BOOST YOUR HEALTH
—— WITH ——
BACTERIA

BOOST YOUR HEALTH
—WITH—
BACTERIA

FRED PESCATORE, MD,
and KAROLYN A. GAZELLA

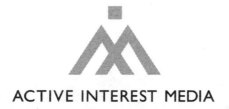

ACTIVE INTEREST MEDIA

Published by:
Active Interest Media, Inc.
300 N. Continental Blvd., Suite 650
El Segundo, CA 90245

Text design by Karen Sperry
Cover design by Silke Design

The information in this book is for educational purposes only and is not recommended as a means of diagnosing or treating an illness. All health matters should be supervised by a qualified healthcare professional. The publisher and the author(s) are not responsible for individuals who choose to self-diagnose and/or self-treat.

Library of Congress Cataloging-in-Publication Data
Pescatore, Fred
Boost Your Health With Bacteria / Fred Pescatore and Karolyn A. Gazella
Includes bibliographical references and index.
1. Health 2. Alternative Medicine 3. Probiotics 4. Bacteria 5. Gazella, Karolyn A
6. Title

ISSN: 978-1-935297-21-5

Printed in the United States of America

ACKNOWLEDGEMENTS

From Karolyn

There are so many individuals that help create a book such as this. I would like to thank our editor, Kim Erickson; our publisher Joanna Shirk; the general manager of the Natural Living Division of Active Interest Media, Pat Fox; and our designers, Karen Sperry and Silke Ruethlinger. I would also like to thank the talented researchers and healthcare professionals we interviewed for the book and a special thank you to Michael Schoor of Essential Formulas Incorporated and the entire Essential Formulas team for supporting this project.

From Dr. Pescatore

I would like to thank many people, but mostly my patients. They are like a family to me and give me strength and motivation to continue to seek out the most cutting edge information. They keep me on my toes at all times and for that I am most grateful. I would also like to thank my family—they know who they are. My inspirations, hopes, dreams, and desires stem from their presence in my life, wherever I may be. I love you!

Also by Fred Pescatore, MD:
>   *Feed Your Kids Well*
>   *Thin For Good*
>   *The Allergy and Asthma Cure*
>   *The Hamptons Diet*
>   *The Hamptons Diet Cookbook*

Also by Karolyn A. Gazella:
>   *Definitive Guide to Cancer*
>   *Return to Beautiful Skin*

PLEASE NOTE

The information in this book reflects the experience of the authors and is not intended to take the place of advice from your own physician. The information is for educational purposes only and is not recommended as a means of diagnosing or treating an illness. All health matters should be supervised by a qualified healthcare professional. You should never attempt to decrease your use of prescription medication without first consulting with your physician. You should also inform your physician of any dietary supplements you are taking. The publisher and the authors are not responsible for individuals who choose to self-diagnose, self-treat or use the information in this booklet without consulting with their own personal health care practitioner.

CONTENTS

Foreword *by Ann Louise Gittleman, PhD, CNS* . . . XI

Introduction 1

PART ONE BATHED IN BACTERIA

CHAPTER 1 Historical Perspective 7

CHAPTER 2 Bacteria Basics 27

CHAPTER 3 Microbial Monsters 45

CHAPTER 4 Friends Forever 57

PART TWO REPOPULATE PROPERLY

CHAPTER 5 Probiotic Pals 73

CHAPTER 6 Going Beyond Probiotics 87

CHAPTER 7 Future of Probiotics 97

PART THREE SOMETHING'S WRONG

CHAPTER 8 Digestion, Elimination, and Detoxification 115

CHAPTER 9 Causes of Illness 129

CHAPTER 10 Specific Conditions 143

PART FOUR BACTERIAL BALANCE

CHAPTER 11 Prevention Plus 193

APPENDIX Terms to Know 213

Selected References 217

Index 229

FOREWORD

THROUGHOUT MY CAREER, I HAVE searched for innovative and effective ways to help people lose weight and detoxify from the toxic world we live in. So I stand in great admiration of forward thinking and visionary health care advocates. That's why I am thrilled to introduce you to this book, *Boost Your Health With Bacteria*. I have personally worked with both authors, Fred Pescatore, MD, a compassionate clinician and best-selling author, and Karolyn A. Gazella, a seasoned and respected health writer.

We now know that the human body is made up of a great deal more bacteria than human cells. As a healthcare professional, I have always been fascinated with bacteria. Understanding both good and bad bacteria is absolutely critical to the health and wellbeing of our nation. In this book, you will learn how enhancing proper bacterial balance can prevent and even treat nearly every major illness of our time. In laymen's terms, the authors take the fascinating topic of bacteria to an entirely new level. They succinctly provide practical information we can use to employ beneficial bacteria and a lifestyle that supports proper bacterial balance in our fight to be healthy and vibrant.

The authors took great measures to be thorough in providing cutting-edge information about bacteria. Experts from the World

Gastroenterology Association and the National Institutes of Health were sought out to provide the most current scientific facts possible. Details about the Human Microbiome Project are provided. This is perhaps one of the most significant international scientific projects undertaken since the Human Genome Project, which identified genes in human DNA. The Human Microbiome Project is determined to make sense of the 100 trillion bacteria housed in the human body. The authors make a compelling case that many of these bacteria can be our "best friends" in preventing disease and healing from serious illness.

In large part, our bacterial make-up dictates if we are to be sick or well. We have always known that bacteria are intimately linked to our digestive system; however, the authors describe in detail how bacteria are connected to immunity and inflammation as well. The authors also cite new scientific research linking bacteria to depression and anxiety, and even weight loss. Bacteria influence our health, literary from head to toe. This book empowers readers to take control of their bacterial balance and, as a result, it will help them take control of their health.

Boost Your Health With Bacteria is comprehensive, easy to understand, and practical. It is a must-read for anyone who is interested in obtaining optimum health and vitality in a world teeming with good and bad bacteria.

Ann Louise Gittleman, PhD, CNS
Author of The Gut Flush Plan

INTRODUCTION

WE ADMIT THIS IS NOT a glamorous subject. To some people, bacteria are frightening or even offensive. While at times they may be just that, they are also incredibly misunderstood. In fact, our publisher highly recommended we not use the word bacteria in the title of this book. Although we made a valiant effort, we could not convey our message without using the word bacteria. There's no denying it, this is a book about bacteria.

This is a life-altering topic and bacteria, in one form or another, are often in the news. Much has been written about why kids should eat dirt (filled with bacteria) and how dangerous our sanitized society (a lack of bacteria) has become. It's difficult to watch television without seeing a commercial that touts the digestive benefits of yogurt (yet another source of bacteria). After discovering that the human body is made up of about 90 percent bacteria and 10 percent human cells, the scientific community has, not surprisingly, become increasingly intrigued by bacteria. The fact is, we are more bacterial than we are human!

The average adult has about 100 trillion bacteria in their body. It only seems logical that such a massive amount of bacteria can influence our health and that there must be bacteria that are on our side. If all of those bacteria were harmful, we'd be dead. The human body is actually designed to have a higher percentage of beneficial bacteria than bad bacteria. The sole purpose of the legions of beneficial bacteria housed in the human body is to keep us healthy—billions of best friends working tirelessly on our behalf. Twitter, Facebook, LinkedIn, and MySpace all pale in comparison to this internal social network. This batch of friends will help determine if you get sick or if you feel well.

The research literature is rife with documentation regarding the broad range of influences that beneficial bacteria have on our health and wellbeing. Your bacterial milieu may even dictate if you are happy or sad, fat or thin, healthy or sick. As a result, beneficial bacteria have also become big business, making it one of the fastest growing categories in the functional food sector. Numerous bacterial products are presently in development including straws laced with beneficial bacteria, bacterial boosts in butter, and even ice cream and chocolate containing our beneficial buddies.

Bacteria are no longer relegated to the back seat. They have become the stars of scientific literature. But before you jump on the bacterial bandwagon, it's important you become informed about your new best friends.

This book takes the pioneering position that beneficial bacteria form the bedrock of good health. In addition to our own investigation, we interviewed experts from around the world including Eamonn Quigley, MD, professor of medicine and physiology at the University College Cork in Cork, Ireland, Alan Krensky, MD, with the National Institutes of Health, and distinguished professor and Japanese research scientist Iichiroh Ohhira, PhD.

Beneficial bacteria can help you prevent disease and, if you are struggling with an illness, they can help you treat it. Just as you focus on important vitamins and minerals in your diet and dietary supplements, you should also focus on beneficial bacteria—perhaps even more.

Bacterial imbalance can be linked to most major illness of our time. Even vague symptoms such as fatigue, anxiety, and weakness can be traced back to improper bacterial balance. In this book, you will learn the role bacteria plays in our everyday lives and how to harness the power of beneficial bacteria to boost your health.

PART ONE
BATHED IN BACTERIA

1

HISTORICAL PERSPECTIVE

PERHAPS YOU'VE HEARD THE SAYING "you are born alone and you die alone." Nothing could be further from the truth. Actually, we are *never* alone. We are constantly and forever surrounded by and bathed in bacteria. Since the dawn of time, humans have shared their existence and their bodies with bacteria. Does that thought give you the creeps? Fear not, because bacteria are not all bad. In fact, most of the bacteria in your body can be considered your best friends.

We will show you how healthy bacteria are actually the missing link to disease prevention, treatment, and ultimately, vibrant health and vitality. Today, there are lots of things we can do to try to be healthy and happy. However, if those healthy bugs are not a part of the battle plan, we will most likely continue to struggle. We are fortunate enough to have billions of best friends we can employ to help us achieve our health goals, no matter what those goals may be. Do you want to lose weight? Are you trying to alleviate uncomfortable symptoms? Do you have a family history of a serious illness such as cancer or heart disease? If the answer is yes to any one of these questions, you need to get to know your bacterial buddies. It may be an unimaginable pairing but it's true, the bacteria living in our bodies are here to help.

Our fear of bad bugs and lack of information about good bugs has led to an onslaught of antibiotic drugs. While these drugs have saved countless lives, they have also become a huge part of the problem because they not only kill the bad bugs, they also kill billions of friendly bacteria that help create and maintain optimum health. Without these billions of good bacteria, our health is in jeopardy. All good bacteria play a significant role in disease prevention and progression. Modern science is now only beginning to understand their significance to our health. The sheer volume makes it impossible for bacteria not to profoundly influence our health. There are far more bacterial cells in the human body than human cells. Their genetics alone outnumber ours by 1,000 times. Bacteria have also been around for billions of years, long before humans ever inhabited this earth, and will probably be around long after we're gone.

Dutch discovery

After scrutinizing fossil remains in rocks, scientists learned that the first bacterium probably inhabited the Earth about 3.5 billion years ago. However, it wasn't until the 1600s when living bacteria were actually observed for the first time.

You would think the most brilliant, highly educated scientist or scientific team available would discover something as significant as bacteria. Surprisingly, that's not the case with this discovery. The unassuming hero of the world of bacteriology (the study of bacteria) was born in 1632 and hailed from the little city of Delft in South Holland, the Netherlands. Antony van Leeuwenhoek was not a scientist at all. He was a curious tradesman with no higher education or university degree, no fortune, and no ties to the scientific community. But van Leeuwenhoek had what it takes to make history—persistence.

At first it appeared van Leeuwenhoek was destined to follow in the family footsteps. There were brewers on his mother's side and his father was a basket maker. After a diverse and varied career working as a fabric merchant, surveyor, and wine assayer, he landed a job grinding lenses to make simple microscopes. His curiosity continued to get the best of him as he began using the microscopes he made. With a microscope that he made himself, van Leeuwenhoek discovered the first bacterium. Starting in 1673, he spent the next 50 years of his life writing to the Royal Society and telling them of his various discoveries—microscopic organisms on bee stings, lake water, and even the plaque between his own teeth.

His descriptions were vivid. At first he called the structures "little animals" and then adopted the term "animalcules." His work was translated and printed in the Philosophical Transactions of the Royal Society. In one description he wrote: "I must have seen quite 20 of these little animals on their long tails alongside one another very gently moving, with outstretched bodies and straightened-out tails; yet in an instant, as it were, they pulled their bodies and their tails together, and no sooner had they contracted their bodies and tails, than they began to stick their tails out again very leisurely, and stayed thus some time continuing their gentle motion."

In 1680, the modest tradesman from Delft, Holland, was made a full member of the Royal Society alongside the most brilliant scientists of his day. Upon his death in 1723, the pastor of his church wrote a letter to the Royal Society commending van Leeuwenhoek's curiosity, craftsmanship, and diligence as he "discovered many secrets of Nature, now famous."

It wasn't until 1838 that the term *bacterium* was introduced by German scientist Christian Gottfried Ehrenberg. The Greek origin of the word bacterium means "small staff"—staff as in stick or rod, not team of employees. Bacteria are the plural form of bacterium. Bacteria like to be surrounded by their friends.

Family history

After van Leewenhoek worked his magic for decades and hard-working scientist Gottfried Ehrenberg nailed down the terminology, the curiosity of the entire scientific community was officially piqued. Over the next 100 or so years, bacteria would receive much-needed attention, with a special focus on the bad bugs.

If you do a quick inventory of the history of bacteria, there are some memorable characters. Most notorious was the deadly bubonic plague of the 1300s that was caused by a type of bacteria known as *Yersinia pestis*. The three-year epidemic took the lives of as many as 50 percent of the European population. Another infamous bacterium, *Mycobacterium leprae*—commonly known as leprosy—has caused pain, suffering, and heartache throughout the ages dating back to first century B.C.

Understandably, scientists were desperate to battle the bad bacteria. Better microscopes were born and scientific techniques were honed for the fight. Numerous discoveries of important bacterial family members followed including:

- 1874 *Streptococcus pyogenes*: strep throat infection
- 1880 *Staphylococcus aureus*: staph infection
- 1885 *Salmonella*: food poisoning
- 1885 *Escherichia coli*: commonly referred to as E. coli
- 1897 *Clostridium botulinum*: botulism
- 1960 *Listeria monocytogenes*: typically found in water
- 1976 *Legionella pneumophila*: Legionnaire's disease
- 1976 *Vibrio vulnificus* from the cholera family: food poisoning from seafood

As you can see, the 1800s were an especially busy time for bacteriologists. Cholera, the most deadly bacteria of all, also entered the picture during that time. According to the Centers for Disease Control and Prevention (CDC), since cholera was discovered there have been a total of seven different widespread cholera attacks called pandemics, the last one in 1961 in Indonesia. A pandemic is described as a widespread outbreak that affects an entire region, continent, or the world. The cholera bacterium is transmitted through food and water.

> *"Chance favors only the prepared mind."*
>
> —*Louis Jean Pasteur*

The list of infamous characters continues to grow even today. As we fast-forward this history lesson, we find even more bacteria with names too long and difficult to pronounce. Most notably is the "super-bug" *methicillin-resistant staphylococcus aureus* (MRSA). Sound familiar? Yes, this one is related to the dreaded staph family. By the way, you'll learn more about superbugs later.

The 1800s introduced more than just famous bacteria. It was during this time that a soon-to-be famous French chemist was born. Louis Jean Pasteur would prove to be one of the most brilliant and famous scientists of our time. In fact, he was one of the founders of the field of microbiology (the study of microbes).

Germ theory

Who knows what exactly motivated Pasteur to save people from infectious diseases? We do know, however, that three of his five children—age two, nine and 13—died of typhoid fever, strong motivation for a brilliant scientist such as Pasteur.

From ancient times throughout the Middle Ages, it was observed that some life forms arose spontaneously from living matter, primarily when something was decaying. This was known as spontaneous generation—the idea that maggots, for example, just occurred spontaneously in rotting meat. Of course, it was later discovered that maggots grew from eggs laid by flies—nothing spontaneous about that.

For Pasteur, it was alcohol, not meat that provided his scientific backdrop. When asked to evaluate some contaminated alcohol, Pasteur found that fermentation was a biologically active process carried out by microorganisms. This finally dismissed the spontaneous generation view and led to the "germ theory"—microorganisms cause infectious diseases. This was a significant historical medical turning point.

Thanks to the germ theory, important discoveries were made in pasteurization (named after Louis himself), antiseptic operations, and contagious diseases. Pasteur believed that if germs could cause fermentation, which in many instances is a positive thing, they could certainly cause contagious diseases. And he was right. This led to his discovery of vaccines.

Not surprisingly, in his day, Pasteur was met with a great deal of resistance. Today, however, germ theory is a cornerstone of clinical microbiology. It has lead to important advances in the area of antibiotics and hospital hygiene practices. In 1895, seven years after he founded the famed Pasteur Institute, Louis Jean Pasteur died.

One of Pasteur's most famous protégés was Nobel-Prize winning scientist Elie Metchnikoff, who eventually became the director of the Pasteur Institute. Metchnikoff was most interested in how bacteria influenced the immune system. His 1908 Nobel Prize was for the discovery of phagocytosis, which is when immune system cells engulf foreign invaders such as bacteria. It was also Metchnikoff who first developed a theory that lactic acid bacteria in the digestive tract could prolong life. This was the first hint that not all bacteria are bad.

Numerous scientists have continued Pasteur and Metchnikoff's work. In the area of treating infectious diseases, the most well known person is Scottish scientist Sir Alexander Fleming, who discovered penicillin in 1928. Taken from mold, penicillin was the first antibiotic discovered and, even today, continues to be one of the most commonly prescribed antibiotic drugs.

Antibiotic onslaught

Sir Alexander Fleming was working on a project with *staphylococci* bacteria when he decided to go on vacation. Upon his return, he found mold growing on the petri dish. As he examined the growth more closely, he realized that there were no staph bacteria growing where the mold was. Not only does this prove that one should periodically take a vacation, it also set in motion the search for the next, more powerful antibiotic.

At the time, Fleming could not have predicted that bacteria are so smart that they would eventually find a way to become resistant to his new-found cure. Soon after its introduction, penicillin had no effect on certain strains of staph. Less than a decade later, there was a whole new class of bacteria killers called sulfonamides.

During the 1940s and early 50s, even more antibiotic drugs were created including streptomycin, chloramphenicol, and tetracycline. The same thing that happened with penicillin happened with these drugs as well—resistance. A trend had developed that continues today: A new antibiotic star hits the market, quickly loses its shine because of resistance, and then there is a mad scramble to find a replacement drug.

Today, antibiotics are one of the most widely prescribed class of drugs in the world. In the United States, they account for more than 12 percent of the prescriptions written and worldwide sales top $23 billion a year.

Although penicillin drugs, specifically amoxicillin, remain the most commonly prescribed type of antibiotic, allergic reactions are common. For individuals who are allergic to penicillins, doctors can choose from more than 100 other antibiotics.

There is no question that antibiotics have saved numerous lives. But in our desperate and zealous attempts to kill bad bacteria, have we created a double-edged sword that has dangerous ramifications no matter which way we swing it? We need antibiotics, and yet their use is helping to create resistant, more virulent and deadly strains of bacteria.

Antibiotic resistance

An antibiotic is chosen based on the type of harmful bacteria present. Often the physician doesn't know exactly which bacterium is causing the problem, so he/she chooses a broad-spectrum antibiotic because it has activity against a wide range of bacteria. Broad-spectrum antibiotics are considered the "big guns" of bacterial warfare. You've probably even been on some of them, like tetracycline or Cipro.

Several reports in the medical literature demonstrate that many antibiotics are misused and overused by the medical community. According to a 2003 *Journal of the American Medical Association* report, broad-spectrum antibiotics were prescribed for the common cold more than 50 percent of the time. And yet, these antibiotics have no affect on the common cold (which is almost always caused by a virus), further leading to antibiotic resistance.

"Microbes exposed to antibiotics evolve dozens of biochemical tricks to inactivate or evade them, and then can pass the tricks around on fragments of DNA," explains Abigail Zugler, MD, in an article she wrote for the *New York Times*. "What is new is the emerging consensus that the way to combat antibiotic resistance may not be bigger, better, stronger antibiotics but, rather, no antibiotics at all."

Research has confirmed that antibiotics can severely disrupt bacterial balance by killing our good bugs as they attempt to kill the bad. Antibiotic use can cause a wide range of unpleasant side effects including:

- soft stools or diarrhea,
- upset stomach,
- vomiting,
- abdominal cramping, and
- vaginal itching or discharge.

Rare but serious side effects to antibiotics can include:

- kidney stones,
- abnormal blood clotting,
- sun sensitivity,
- blood disorders, and
- deafness.

Jessica Snyder Sachs writes in her book, *Good Germs, Bad Germs*, that antibiotics, especially broad-spectrum antibiotics, "frequently trigger 'yeast' infections (caused by the fungus *Candida albicans*), bacterial vaginosis (caused by an imbalance of intestinal bacteria), or a maddening cycle of one followed by the other." Antibiotics disrupt the ecological balance of our internal bacteria because they kill all bacteria—bad and good alike. Their overuse can be dangerous on many levels.

Superheroes versus superbugs

While antibiotics have saved millions of lives, surveys conducted by the CDC confirm there is a serious problem of the misuse and overuse of prescription antibiotics. As a result, we have managed to create new, more virulent strains of bacteria that are not only difficult to treat, they can be deadly. Bacteria that have several resistant genes are called superbugs. Superbugs are drug-resistant and primarily exist as a result of the overuse of antibiotics.

A 2001 report featured in the journal *American Family Physician* reported that as many as 50 percent of the antibiotic prescriptions written were believed to be unnecessary, a trend that continues today. According to the report, 90 to 95 percent of all sore throats are not bacterially based, and yet doctors still prescribe antibiotics in many of those cases.

Antibiotics also find their way into our food and water supply. An investigation by Associated Press journalists Jeff Donn, Martha Mendoza, and Justin Pritchard discovered that antibiotics, as well as many other pharmaceuticals, were in the drinking water that supplied at least 41 million Americans.

The Union of Concerned Scientists, a consumer advocacy group, has estimated that nearly 25 million pounds of antibiotics are used in the United States livestock industry each year, which is more than eight times the amount of antibiotics used in human medicine. Contrary to the United States, the European Union completed an aggressive six-year plan that phased out antibiotics as growth promoters in their livestock industry. When we ingest the meat of these animals, we are ingesting antibiotics without even knowing it.

"Over the last 30 years, scores of studies have confirmed that this steady diet of antibiotics breeds highly resistant microflora in an animal's digestive tract and on its skin, as well as in the air, soil, and groundwater in and around livestock operations," explains Sachs. The dangerous rise of the virulent strain of *Escherichia coli (E. coli)* 0157 that has plagued our beef, poultry, and produce industry can be attributed directly to antibiotics in the food chain. While we often think of *E. coli* affecting the meat industry, outbreaks in produce have been found because of runoff from nearby livestock facilities. *E. coli* was a harmless inhabitant of the digestive tract in most humans until it developed resistance to antibiotics just a few short years ago.

The rise of antibiotic-resistant infections has been spreading fast. The *New England Journal of Medicine* reported in 1994 that researchers had already identified bacteria in patient samples that resisted all

Antibiotics have saved countless lives. But according to Stuart B. Levy, MD, of Tufts University School of Medicine, their misuse and overuse for viral illnesses and in animals is "wasting good products and creating this resistance, which comes back to everyone in society, those that take the antibiotics and those that don't."

The Difference Between Bacteria And Viruses

The definition of bacteria is single-cell microorganisms that can live on their own. Some bacteria can cause disease. Antibiotics can kill bacteria.

Viruses, on the other hand, are defined as microscopic infectious agents that are unable to live outside a host. Viruses cannot be killed by antibiotics.

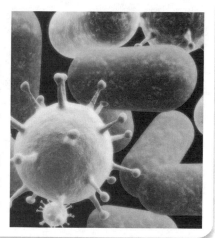

currently available antibiotic drugs. In just one short decade, from the early 1980s to the early 1990s, resistance to penicillin by pneumonia bacterial strains jumped from .02 percent to nearly seven percent.

Also in the early 1990s, the *New England Journal of Medicine* reported that a newly recognized strain of *Clostridium difficile (C. diff)* bacteria caused an epidemic of diarrhea in various hospitals throughout the United States. Researchers found that the *C. diff* strain was highly resistant to the antibiotic clindamycin, stating that using clindamycin significantly increases the risk of severe diarrhea. A significant number of children have *C. diff* naturally present in the gut. This bacterium typically does not cause problems; however, in some cases when antibiotics are used to treat other illnesses, the *C. diff* bacteria can multiply and cause diarrhea. *C. diff* is highly contagious and, in some cases, can be deadly. Good hygiene practices in the hospital setting is the best way to prevent *C. diff* infections.

Antibiotic use for acne is also problematic. A study completed by researcher David J. Margolis, MD, PhD, and his colleagues at the University of Pennsylvania Center for Education and Research in Therapeutics, demonstrated that individuals who took antibiotics long-term for their acne had a two-fold increase in upper respiratory

The Swine Flu Virus

In Spring 2009, the world braced itself for a possible viral pandemic as the Swine Flu infected the country of Mexico. Soon, the virus was top of mind as more cases were diagnosed in other countries, including the United States. There are a number of things to focus on when trying to prevent the spread of a deadly virus such as the Swine Flu including the following:

Frequent hand washing is imperative. In the case of children, wash the hands of young children and remind older children of the necessity to wash their hands thoroughly and often.

Try to bolster your health and the health of your immune system through diet, dietary supplements, stress reduction, being physically active, getting enough sleep, and drinking plenty of liquids.

Avoid close contact with people who are sick.

Avoid contact with surfaces and items that may be contaminated, such as desks, tables, water bottles, etc.

Cover your nose and mouth with a tissue when you cough or sneeze and then quickly throw out the tissue and wash your hands thoroughly.

Germs spread when you touch your eyes, nose, or mouth so avoid touching these areas unless your hands are washed thoroughly.

If you feel sick, you should stay home and avoid contact with others.

The most common way for these types of illnesses to spread is by having the droplets from a cough or sneeze land on a surface and then have another individual touch that surface and then touch their mouth, nose, or eyes before washing their hands. Viruses can live on surfaces for two hours or longer. The CDC warns that these viruses can be spread even before symptoms are present. In the case of the swine flu, an individual can be contagious for seven or more days after onset. Small children tend to be contagious for longer periods of time.

If you are concerned about your flu symptoms, seek medical care.

tract infections. In a previous study, Dr. Margolis found an association between antibiotic use and an increase in strep throat infections.

A highly resistant strain of staph bacteria previously thought to be problematic only in hospitals has now made its way into our communities. A 2007 report from the CDC indicates that methicillin-resistant *staphylococcus aureus* (MRSA) kills more people each year than AIDS. It is believed that MRSA-related deaths are even higher than present estimates because MRSA can cause heart, liver, or kidney failure or pneumonia, which is often listed as the cause of death. The MRSA bacteria create a toxic protein that destroys tissue as it grows rapidly. Media reports about MRSA infection have become common-place. Remember, the MRSA bug grew up in what is supposed to be the most sanitary place we can go, the hospital.

Stuart B. Levy, MD, of Tufts University School of Medicine, told CNN in 2000, "We have patients in the United States dying from infections that are untreatable. This is unthinkable."

Evidence also suggests that antibiotic use can increase the risk of breast cancer in susceptible women. According to Dr. Levy, while the initial findings do not demonstrate a direct cause and effect, it is important to find out why there is an association between increased antibiotic use and breast cancer. One answer is that antibiotic use can weaken the immune system and our ability to control inflammation, both of which can lead to serious illnesses including cancer and heart disease.

As we learn more about bacteria, it is important to understand the difference between bacteria and viruses. Clarification is vital if we are to reduce antibiotic resistance, especially in cases of illnesses mostly caused by viruses such as the common cold.

Virus versus bacteria

There is often confusion regarding the difference between viruses and bacteria. Some people believe that influenza (a.k.a. the flu) is

Getting to Know Harmful Bacteria

Name	Description
Bacillus anthracis	Causes a deadly disease in cattle known as anthrax and can also be used as a potential bioweapon against humans.
Brucella abortus	Causes an infectious disease among livestock and is primarily passed among animals, but humans can also become infected.
Clostridium botulinum	Referred to as botulism, this bacterium is a nerve toxin that can cause paralysis.
Escherichia coli	The most well-known bacteria, it is also the most common bacteria living in the gut; the "bad" strain of E. coli O157:H7 causes severe food borne sickness; E. coli is also linked to ulcers and stomach cancer.
Legionella pneumophilla	This bacterium was discovered in 1976 after a mysterious deadly pneumonia outbreak. Because it first appeared at an American Legion convention, the illness it caused was dubbed Legionnaires disease.
Mycobacterium tuberculosis	Causes tuberculosis, an infectious disease that typically attacks the lungs and can also damage other parts of the body.
Salmonella	A group of bacteria usually passed from the feces of people or animals that cause one of the most common intestinal infections in the United States is called salmonellosis (a.k.a. food poisoning).
Salmonella typhi	This is a specific virulent salmonella bacterium that is responsible for causing typhoid fever. This bacterium is spread via food or water that has been contaminated by someone who is carrying the *salmonella typhi* bacteria.
Staphylococcus	Also known as staph, this is one of the most dangerous drug-resistant bacteria. It can cause serious, even deadly, infections.
Streptococcus pneumoniae	Causes "strep" throat, tonsillitis, meningitis, and pneumonia.
Vibrio cholerae	Commonly referred to as cholera, this bacterium is deadly and can be transmitted through fecally-contaminated water or food.

a bacterial infection when, in fact, it is a virus. The common cold is also a virus. Taking an antibiotic is not necessary in these situations. One symptom of the common cold can be a sore throat. Sometimes the *streptococcus* bacterium is the cause of a sore throat—also referred to as strep throat. Strep throat is a bacterial infection unrelated to cold and flu viruses. If a physician believes you may have strep throat, she/he will test for the presence of bacteria in the throat. If strep bacteria are found, the physician will most likely prescribe an antibiotic.

According to Bill Bryson author of *A Short History of Nearly Everything*, in isolation, viruses are harmless. He says they "prosper by hijacking the genetic material of a living cell and using it to produce more viruses. They reproduce fanatically and burst out in search of more cells to invade."

Viruses and bacteria have many differences but the most critical one is that a virus will not respond to antibiotic treatment, whereas bacteria can be killed by an antibiotic.

Doctors aren't the only ones to blame for the overuse of antibiotics. Physicians, in particular emergency room physicians, are often faced with patients who demand a prescription for an antibiotic. According to emergency room physician Susan Ryan, DO, it can be difficult for patients to understand that they don't need an antibiotic. What typically distinguishes a cold virus from influenza are a fever, a more prominent headache, much more severe aches and pains, and very disabling fatigue and weakness. But even with those horrible symptoms, a cold and flu are viral and will not respond to antibiotics. The same is true for a nasty cough that is not caused by the strep bacteria or lung congestion that is not caused by pneumonia. "If strep is not present and the lungs are clear, it is not caused by bacteria and will not respond to antibiotic treatment," explains Dr. Ryan, who is with Rose Emergency in Denver, CO. She says she tries to explain to patients that a virus simply needs to run its course and will clear in seven to 14 days. She gets frustrated that even after her explanation, some patients continue to want a prescription for an antibiotic. No matter how badly you feel, avoid the temptation to pressure your doctor into prescribing an antibiotic.

Germ killing spree

Our fear of bacteria has become obsessive. Not only are we using a bomb-shell approach with antibiotic treatment, we employ countless germ-killing products to scorch, cleanse, and sanitize our homes, hospitals, and bodies, in a desperate—and ill-advised—attempt to rid our world of these insidious beastly bugs. In the process, we have made them stronger.

Let's use MRSA as our example. Years ago, when doctors found that penicillin was not affective on some staph infections due to a built up resistance, they started using methicillin. Eventually, the staph became resistant to this drug also and voila, methicillin-resistant *staph aureus*. This bacterium is so powerful it is labeled a "superbug" because it is resistant to several different antibiotics—even the drug designed to originally treat it. Previously only found in hospitals, MRSA has now infiltrated our communities. While MRSA has been around for decades, it has only recently been successful at making its way to the general public.

One of the most common news stories about MRSA is the athlete that has inadvertently snatched it up while working out. Outbreaks have been reported in major universities, professional team locker rooms, and even at the high school level. As a result, trainers desperately, obsessively, and understandably wipe down equipment with disinfectant products. It's been a boon for the microbial products industry. According to a *Newsweek* feature, in 2007 alone there were about 200 different antimicrobial products introduced into the market. But is this the answer? Should we blast

Natural Alternatives to Antibiotics

With issues of antibiotic resistance becoming more prevalent, it's worth exploring natural alternatives to these drugs. While natural substances cannot completely replace antibiotics, some herbs can provide viable options in mild bacterial infections and also in many minor viral infections such as a cold or the flu. The two most commonly used and widely studied herbs with antibiotic activity are goldenseal and garlic.

The three main active alkaloids in goldenseal that have been shown to have antibiotic activity are berberine, hydrastine, and canadine. The antibiotic effects of these alkaloids are well documented in the scientific literature. In particular, berberine has been shown to be effective against a wide range of harmful organisms including: *Staphylococcal sp, Streptococcus sp., Chlamydia sp., Corynebacterium diphtheria, Salmonella typhi, Vibrio cholerae, Diplococcus pneumonia,* and *Candida albicans.*

Aged garlic extract also has a wide range of antimicrobial activity against many types of bacteria, virus, worms, and fungi. Some studies demonstrate that garlic is more effective than nystatin, gentian violet, and other antifungal agents. Garlic can be especially effective against the *Candida albican* fungus.

According to *Functional Ingredients* magazine, researchers from the University College Cork in Ireland have clearly demonstrated that beneficial bacteria (a.k.a. probiotics) can be used in place of antibiotics to prevent and treat specific illnesses in animals. The researchers speculate that confirmation of probiotics as a first-line of prevention and treatment for bacterial conditions in humans is eminent. "It is likely that using probiotics rather than antibiotics will appeal to at-risk individuals since they are safe, non-invasive, do not create resistance bacteria, and can even be administered in the form of tasty foods and beverages," said Colin Hill, MD, of University College Cork, who presented his findings at the Society for General Microbiology meeting in the United Kingdom on April 2, 2009.

One of the best ways to avoid antibiotics is to have a strong immune system. To bolster your immune system while supporting your friendly bacteria, follow the advice featured in Chapters 4 and 11.

bacteria with antibiotics and then try to suffocate them with germ-killing chemicals?

"Americans have been obsessed with eradicating germs ever since their role in disease was discovered in the 19th century," according to the *Newsweek* report, "but they've been partial to technological fixes like antibiotics and sanitizers rather than the dirty work of cleanliness."

Nobody is saying that we need to stop sanitizing, but going on a germ-killing spree is not the answer. Chapter 2 features important information on precautions you can take to reduce your exposure to dangerous microbes.

Time for a change

History has trained us to think that the only good bacteria are dead bacteria. People think of bacteria as germy, dirty little bugs that cause disease. That's why we've historically employed the big guns—antibiotics—to blast out the nasty microbes from the inside out.

"No one yearns for the days before antibiotics, when doctors could do little more for their feverish patients than wait to see if they survived the night," according to Sachs in *Good Germs, Bad Germs*. "Nor would any reasonable person propose that we trade modern sanitation for the epidemics of cholera, dysentery, typhoid fever, and bubonic plague that began decimating populations with the advent of civilization some five thousand years ago."

We know it's time for a change, but how do we balance on that razor's edge, keeping the technology that has saved so many lives while getting back to basics so we can save countless others. The answer is not to throw out the antibiotics and the antimicrobial sanitation products.

We agree with Sachs who writes, "Clearly, mounting a direct assault on the bacterial kingdom has always been foolhardy, given how rapidly these organisms can evolve around any biochemical weapon we throw at them. Rather than escalate an arms race we can never win, many scientists are now looking for better approaches to the problem."

It's time for a new strategy that begins with the old war adage, "know thy enemy." Since not all bacteria are harmful to us—and many play a beneficial role—we must find out which bacteria are really the enemies.

CHAPTER

2

BACTERIA BASICS

ONE OF THE FIRST THINGS scientists noticed about bacteria is that there are a lot of them. That's clearly an understatement. The human body is made up of a mixture of cells and bacteria. Biologists estimate that bacteria outnumber the cells in the human body by 10 to 1—maybe even 100 to 1. There are about 100 trillion bacteria in the intestinal tract alone. 100 trillion is a lot of bacteria. Can these massive communities of microorganisms actually help us prevent and treat illness?

Bacteria come in three basic shapes: rod, ball, and spiral. When they join together they can look like a cluster of fuzzy circles, a mass of tangled string, or an elegant ribbon. As described in Chapter 1, we are most familiar with the "bad" bacteria that transmit disease. As Metchnikoff discovered, however, there is such a thing as a "good" bacterium. Dietary supplements that resemble, replicate, or provide the same human strains of the good bacteria in the gut are called pro-biotics (i.e. "for life"). By the way, we find it interesting that the literal meaning of antibiotic is "against life."

In addition to the trillions of bacteria housed in the human body, bacteria live on or in virtually every type of material found on earth. A mere teaspoon of soil contains more than a billion bacteria. A recent genome study found there are one million bacteria in every square centimeter of the crook of your elbow, and that's not even their favorite hiding place. As you can see, not only are there a lot of them, they are everywhere!

What are they?

Bacteria consist of a single cell and can vary dramatically in size. While the largest known bacterium is big enough to be seen without a microscope, most bacteria are very small and cannot be seen with the naked eye. Millions of bacteria can fit into the eye of a needle. Because of their small size, bacteria are often referred to as microflora. Technically, microflora is any microscopic organism. However, in the case of bacteria in your body, microflora commonly refers to microscopic bacterial colonies living in the intestines.

Bacteria may be tiny in stature, but they certainly pack a powerful punch. According to the American Society for Microbiology (www. MicrobeWorld.org), there is even a strain of bacteria that can withstand blasts of radiation 1,000 times greater than would kill a human. Some bacteria are even able to live in cold that would freeze your blood or heat far above boiling. And they're fast. Bacteria can move at about 50 to 60 body lengths per second. That's equal to a six-foot-tall man running nine times faster than the world record! Bacteria multiply a million times more rapidly than we do.

Bacteria also have a very diverse appetite. Depending on the species, bacteria will eat anything from sugar, starches, sunlight, sewage, wood, and nails; they will even consume us after we die. They can eat what we eat and nearly everything else, too.

A bacterial species is typically defined in terms of resembling characteristics. Within each species, there are subsets called strains. A strain of the same species of bacteria can have some minor identifiable differences. It's critical to know both the species and the strain.

When dealing with bacteria (both friendly and unfriendly), the species and the strain names provide important information. Let's give you a quick example. Different strains of bacteria within the same species can have very different effects. In the case of *Lactobacillus acidophilus* DDS-1, *Lactobacillus* is the genus, *acidophilus* is the species, and DDS-1 is the strain. Another example is *Lactobacillus acidophilus* GG. This is the same genus and species of *Lactobacillus* but it is a different strain. Jerry Adler and Jeneen Interlandi wrote in *Newsweek* that there are thousands of different species inside us, found in numerous combinations as unique as our fingerprint.

Most human bacteria live in the gut, which is the area in the body that spans from the esophagus to the anus. However, there are also bacteria living happily in the mouth, in and around the reproductive organs, groin, and all over the skin. The appendix is also packed with bacteria just waiting to be deployed to the intestines when needed. About 100 billion bacteria make their home on your skin, and there are more than 10 billion bacteria just in your mouth. But that pales in comparison to what people excrete in their feces every day—more than one quadrillion bacteria worldwide!

While bacteria are small single cells, their activity is complex. They are constantly communicating with each other and with our other cells. They also have a powerful influence on our health. It's absolutely critical that we learn everything we can about bacteria.

Bacteria also enjoy a special kinship with each other. Maybe that's why there are so many of them—they like company. "Most bacteria shun the solitary and drifting lifestyle that scientists glimpse in test-tube cultures of a single species," explains Sachs. She says, "In nature they readily organize themselves into diverse communities, divvying up duties from food manufacture to garbage disposal to public defense." In addition to their diverse communities, there are even unique neighborhoods within the same community. Two teeth in the same mouth, for example, can host different bacterial species.

Human Microbiome Project

To help us understand more about the bugs in and on our bodies, in 2007 the National Institutes of Health (NIH) launched the Human Microbiome Project. The Google definition of a microbiome is "the entourage of associated microflora in a host." It appears as though entourages are not just for politicians and actors anymore. According to UC Davis professor Jonathan Eisen, PhD, a microbiome is "the sum collection of all the microbes found in or on people." Dr. Eisen, who is a evolutionary biologist specializing in microbes, says "it seems a no-brainer that there is a need for a coordinated project to gather background information about the human microbiome that would then be useful to researchers, much like the human genome was useful to many researchers."

Just as the human genome project gave us valuable information about different genes, the microbiome project will identify and characterize microbial communities living inside and on us. The interesting part of the Human Microbiome Project is that it will evaluate healthy human volunteers, rather than trying to grow various bacteria in a petri dish in the laboratory. This allows scientists to observe bacteria in their natural habitat. According to the NIH, samples will be collected from five body regions that are viewed as favorite resting spots for many microbes. This includes the digestive tract, mouth, skin, nose, and female urogenital tract.

"I am extremely enthusiastic about the Human Microbiome Project as it promises to reveal the true magnitude and diversity of the human microbiota which has been grossly underestimated by conventional culture techniques," explains Eamonn Quigley, MD, President of the World Gastroenterology Association and professor of medicine at the University College Cork in Ireland.

For decades, researchers have been "growing" bacteria in the lab with the hope of understanding them. This is known as a microbial "culture" (more about this in Part Two). We now know, however, that many of the bacterial strains in the human body can't be grown in isolation. Even if a bacterial representative from a species can be grown in the lab, it doesn't reflect the true diversity of that bacterial population.

Accomplishing the goals of the Microbiome Project won't be easy. "There likely will be enormous variation in and among people," explains Dr. Eisen. "Within a person, there will be variation over time as well as great variation in different sites." For example, recent research from the National Human Genome Research Institute discovered that the type of bacteria residing in the inner elbow are completely different than the bacteria living just a few inches away on the inner forearm.

The NIH is collaborating with many other organizations and other countries. This is a huge investment in both time and money. As part of the NIH's Roadmap for Medical Research, the Human Microbiome Project will award $115 million to researchers over a five-year period.

"Our goal is to discover what microbial communities exist in different parts of the human body and to explore how these communities change in the presence of health and disease," explains Francis S. Collins, MD, PhD, former National Human Genome Research Institute Director and a co-chair of the Human Microbiome Project Implementation Group. Dr. Collins says, "In addition, we will likely identify novel genes and functional elements in microbial genomes that will reshape the way we think about and approach human biology." Alan M. Krensky, MD, Deputy Director for the Office of Portfolio Analysis and Strategic Initiatives with the NIH, was kind enough to provide an update on how the Human Microbiome Project is going (for more information refer to the interview on page 42). Part Two features an in-depth interview with Dr. Krensky.

The NIH admits, "little is known about the role this astounding assortment of bacteria, fungi, and other microbes play in human health and disease." The Human Microbiome Project has already confirmed that we know remarkably little about the complex interactions we have with the bacteria in and on our bodies. The project has already identified over 2,000 types of bacteria on/in the human volunteers. Hopefully, this project will help show us how beneficial microbes contribute to our health. Instead of killing microbes to control infectious disease, the goal is to develop new medicines based on utilizing the healing powers of bacteria. Just as the germ theory was in the 1800s, results from the Human Microbiome Project could prove to be another significant turning point in medical history.

What prompted the Human Microbiome Project in the first place? Weight loss. That's right, bacteria may lead us to our next weight loss wonder. This information not only caught the attention of the NIH, it was big news for the general public as well. The NIH and the European Union were already evaluating the benefits of doing the Human Microbiome Project. However, when Jeffrey Gordon, MD, and his research team from Washington University, found that microbes could make a fat mouse thin and vice versa, the public couldn't get enough of that story. Other researchers jumped on the bandwagon and confirmed Gordon's preliminary results. Imagine if all we had to do to lose weight was to take a few extra probiotic pills? While we all realize that weigh loss is not that simple, it became clear to the NIH and researchers throughout the world that bacteria play a significant role in health and disease. There is even talk that bacteria can make us happy or sad (more on that in Part Three). The Human Microbiome Project is just one of many efforts attempting to illuminate the specific roles bacteria play. The key is to find out how to use that information to enhance health and treat illness.

Listening in

There has been a critical shift in the way researchers look at bacteria. We are now starting to balance our research, hopefully, on both identifying and killing bad bacteria, and on identifying and supporting the good bacteria.

To support the friendly and reduce the unfriendly, we first need to listen to what they are saying. Researchers are finding ways to eavesdrop on the billions of bacterial conversations that take place in the human body. That's right, bacteria talk to each other, and they talk to our other cells as well. But what are they actually saying to each other—and what are they telling our other cells? Researchers are searching for ways to tap into this bacterial chatter so we can understand what's going on and, even more significantly, learn how we can influence these conversations.

Research by Bonnie L. Bassler, PhD, Princeton geneticist and Howard Hughes Medical Institute Investigator, says bacteria actually invented cell-to-cell communication. Dr. Bassler told PBS that if you compare bacterial communication to our words and languages, bacteria are most likely multilingual. For example, one bacterial species may speak English, while another speaks French, she says. And then there is another molecule that speaks a language that everyone can understand, which she calls "the trade language." "One species still can't understand the private language of other species," she told PBS, "but they can all understand the trade language."

Dr. Bassler says bacteria use a chemical language known as quorum sensing in order to communicate. One of the most critical aspects of quorum sensing that she has discovered is that it allows bacteria to count their numbers, develop a critical mass, and then change their behavior in unison to carry out their task. Bacteria, as it turns out, are definitely team players, and they work really well together. Even when an entire colony is nearly wiped out, the one or two lone survivors can quickly communicate, recruit, and adapt. No wonder they are so good at resisting our offenses!

Bacteria are great group communicators, but they also know how to interrupt communication of other cells. According to Dr. Bassler, "We know that different species of bacteria can trick each other and garble up each other's languages." This happens both with bad bacteria and with good bacteria. The key is to enhance communication among good bacteria, while disrupting communication among the bad microbes. Bassler's research is trying to figure out how to keep bad bacteria from talking or at least stop the good bacteria from listening to the bad.

What makes a good communicator? Someone who is strong and healthy. It's hard to communicate effectively when we are feeling tired and outnumbered. The same is true for our friendly bacteria.

Hard at work

As we have learned, not all bacteria are bad. In fact, many bacteria possess incredible healing powers. In addition to their healing touch, our friendly bacteria also crowd out harmful bacteria. Like the old story of the Hatfields and McCoys, bacterial families work hard to protect their space along the intestinal wall. Technically, this is known as "competitive exclusion." We want the good bacteria to win that competition. When our good bacteria are healthy and robust, they can strong-arm their way into every nook and cranny in or on our bodies so when the bad bacteria show up there's simply "no room at the inn." Our good bacteria can then form a protective barrier against invading bad bacteria.

Both good and bad bacteria scope out the territory and settle on the best spot for themselves and their families. And when you notice certain smells coming from your body, that's bad bacteria letting you know they've chosen to live under your arm, between your toes, or in your mouth.

Good bacteria are not as noticeable as the bad, but they are some of the hardest working molecules in the human body. Our friendly bacteria perform a wide range of important tasks that includes:
- helping to digest foods;
- processing and manufacturing important vitamins;
- managing and eliminating toxic substances; and
- killing harmful bacteria.

Good bacteria kill bad bacteria by releasing natural bacteriocins. This is an important part of their sophisticated chemical communication process. In addition, good bacteria can interfere with the communication of bad bacteria, thwarting their efforts to multiple and band together.

As you can see, not all bacteria are self-serving. In many cases, friendly bacteria form important alliances with our other cells, protecting us from harm and ensuring that critical tasks are managed properly. They support a vast array of cells in the immune system, brain, heart, and other key body systems. The fact is, without bacteria, we would be dead.

As Sachs describes it, good bacteria "form a kind of protective mulch that has always been our best defense against infectious disease. The absence of their constant, reassuring touch appears to leave the immune system on hair trigger, with a nasty tendency to shoot up the neighborhood."

Because there are so many bacteria, it's comforting to know that not all of them are bad. In fact, scientists are now discovering that most of the 2,000 strains of bacteria already identified on humans are beneficial. Our bodies are actually designed to have proper bacterial balance with the good outnumbering the bad.

In the first two years of life, our specific internal bacterial recipe—which is as unique as our fingerprint—is determined. The various strains that make up our bacterial blueprint stay with us throughout our entire lives. The only thing that ebbs and flows is the ratio of friendly to unfriendly bacteria. We agree with other clinicians and researchers who have found that a healthy colon should contain a ratio of 85 percent good bacteria to not more than 15 percent bad bacteria.

When we have at least five times more friendly than unfriendly bacteria, our bodies function efficiently and we are symptom-free. When the bad outweighs the good, we feel out of balance, have less energy, and may even put on a few extra pounds. It's during these times of bad bacterial dominance that illness can set it.

Bacterial influences

Most bacteria are stubborn, self-preserving cells intent on duplication and survival. This is good news when the bacteria are our friends— and bad news if they don't have our best interests in mind.

Zugler wrote in the *New York Times* that most bacteria "are industrious and friendly, minding their own business in tight-knit, long-lived communities, doing the grunt biochemical work we depend on to stay alive. A few miscreants, though, will kill us if we let them stay."

Even before we are born, there is a plan in place to protect us from harmful invaders such as bacteria, fungi, parasites, and yeast. While we are still in the womb, friendly bacteria alter the pH of our mother's vagina. This helps protect us from dangerous invaders as we slip through the birth canal. There is a very good reason why we come out head first. "This head-to-anus juxtaposition ensures that, of all the billions of microbes the baby will meet in its first day of life, the first will be those to which its mother's immune system has already developed protective antibodies," writes Sachs.

The womb is a completely sterile environment. A baby's first exposure to beneficial bacteria is through vaginal birth and breast-feeding. Because of this, supplemental probiotics are vital to both mother and infant.

In addition to bolstering a baby's immune system, the billions of bacteria in the human colon serve a variety of important functions including extracting nutrients from our foods while fortifying our defenses against disease-causing foes. Bacteria can even enhance serotonin levels, the feel-good hormone found in the central nervous system. Bacteria influence what we eat and when. For that reason, good bacteria may even help with weight loss. Most

Gauge Your Gut

To determine if you have proper bacterial balance, answer the following questions:

	yes	no
Have you taken an antibiotic within the past 12 months?		
Have you experienced constipation or diarrhea within the past three months?		
Do you experience abdominal cramping a few hours after eating?		
Is abdominal pain relieved after passing gas?		
Do you experience pain during bowel movements?		
Do your abdominal discomforts, constipation and/or diarrhea get worse with stress?		
Arc you frequently bloated?		
Do you experience heart burn or burning in your stomach?		
Do you have trouble losing weight?		
Do you have food allergies?		

If you answered yes to 3 or more of these questions, you most likely have an imbalance of bad to good bacteria.

importantly, bacteria found in the gut help regulate our immune system. If you increase the balance of good to bad bacteria in the intestinal tract, you will positively promote the power of the immune system, our primary means of protection against pathogens, foreign invaders, cancer growth, and disease. Chapter 10 features a detailed list of all the conditions good bacteria may positively influence. That chapter provides condition descriptions and treatment options.

If you look at nearly every key part of the body, you will find harmful bacteria and bacteria-related issues. Here are just a few examples:

- More than 500 different bacterial strains reside in the mouth, many of which can lead to cavities and gingivitis.
- Conjunctivitis (pink eye) can be caused by bacteria.
- When bacteria enter the middle ear, they can cause a painful infection.
- *Propionibacterium* can cause acne.
- In some cases, bacteria can play a role in heart disease.
- Pneumonia is caused by bacteria in the lungs.
- *Helicobacter pylori* bacteria can cause ulcers and even lead to stomach cancer.
- A number of bacteria can cause sexually transmitted diseases.
- Many abdominal and liver infections are caused by bacteria.

Because they are so widespread and they far outnumber our other cells, bacteria can positively or negatively influence our health. We often associate bad bacteria with the colon. That's because initial symptoms of bacterial imbalance often surface as intestinal disturbances including diarrhea, constipation, gas, bloating, cramping, and other bowel discomforts. But the ramifications of these monstrous microbes can be devastating and travel far beyond the bowel.

Out of balance

Have you ever felt a little "off?" This is a common way we describe being out of balance—we feel off. Perhaps it begins with embarrassing gas or uncomfortable bloating, even after we eat a small meal. Or maybe you've noticed poor energy levels or that you get sick more frequently.

Numerous aspects of modern-day living can lead to a dangerous bacterial imbalance with bad bacteria weighing you down,

What happens when bad bugs turn deadly?

There was a time, not that long ago, when bugs were pretty basic. There were good ones and bad ones, and our only mission was to kill the bad ones. However, bacteria are not that simple. As it turns out, bad bacteria are far more "intelligent" than we previously assumed. For example, the deadly *E. coli* bacterium has inhabited the human stomach for centuries. In turned deadly just a few decades ago and, in certain people, can cause ulcers and even stomach cancer. The bacteria *Legionella pneumophila* has also been around for centuries—and yet it only surfaced as a deadly bug in 1976 after attendees at an American Legion conference were exposed to it through aerosolized water droplets from the air conditioning system. It is the cause of the notorious outbreak known as Legionnaire's disease. The same is true for the strain of *staphylococcus aureus* that became resistant to methicillin antibiotic. This super bug, known simply as MRSA, was once confined to hospitals and long-term care facilities but has now seeped out into our communities. In 2007, the CDC reported that MRSA has become "a major public health problem."

taking over, and causing all kinds of symptoms. A variety of factors can tip the scales in favor of the harmful bacteria, including:

- overuse and misuse of antibiotics;
- use of steroidal medications and/or oral contraceptives;
- excess stress;
- poor nutrition;
- lack of physical activity;
- overuse of antimicrobial products; and
- serious illness.

All of these factors weaken our immune system, increase inflammation, and kill our good bacteria. This provides many opportunities for the bad bacteria to secure their foothold and establish their turf. For example, poor nutrition means we are not eating enough good bacteria to repopulate and replenish our friendly bacterial colonies.

Chapters 4 and 11 provide specific ways to support good bacteria through diet and lifestyle.

When the bad bacteria outnumber the good, the resulting imbalance—also known as *dysbiosis*—can lead to a whole host of problems including digestive disorders, vaginitis, high cholesterol, heart disease, and cancer. Part Three has a lot more information on the variety of conditions that can result from a negative bacterial balance of more bad than good. Bacterial imbalance is diagnosed by looking at health history, symptoms, and stool samples. In some cases, more involved tests such as a colonoscopy or ultrasound may be required. We'll go into more detail about the signs and symptoms of bacterial imbalance in the next chapter.

The key to correcting bacterial imbalance is to understand our link with both the good and bad bacteria, and learn how they interact with each other and with our other cells. "Only by understanding the symbiotic aspects of our long-standing relationship with microbes can we find lasting solutions to infectious disease and, at the same time, rectify the imbalances that have produced a modern epidemic of allergies, autoimmune disorders, and other inflammatory diseases," Sachs explains. This concept is part of the new paradigm of probiotic medicine.

Bacteria help the immune system develop. Some researchers believe that our lack of exposure to bad bugs, as well as the overuse of antibiotics, has undermined the crucial bacterial element in immunity and contributed to a dramatic increase in allergies, asthma, and autoimmune disorders such as lupus and multiple sclerosis.

Bacteria directly communicate with the B and T cells of the immune system. When antibiotics or the other lifestyle factors listed previously negatively influence our good bacteria, the immune cells don't receive their signal, resulting in a breakdown in immune activity. It's as if the bad bacteria cut the telephone lines between the good

Why organic?

In the United States, the livestock industry routinely uses antibiotics for growth production or as prevention. These antibiotics eventually make their way into our bodies. "Analyses of supermarket meat and eggs show that at least some of this drug-resistant microflora also ends up shrink-wrapped with the meat we buy and trapped inside eggs before their shells form," explains Jessica Snyder Sachs in her book *Good Germs, Bad Germs*.

What can you do? Buy organic. What does it mean to buy organic meat and poultry? According to the Organic Trade Association, it means the animals:
- cannot be given antibiotics or growth hormones;
- are fed 100 percent organic feed;
- have access to the outdoors, fresh air, water, sunshine, grass and pastures; and
- have shelter that allows them an opportunity to exercise.

Organic practices are not only better for the animal, they are better for the environment and for our health. It's true that the organic industry is not perfect. For example, chickens and cows should be eating the food they were meant to eat, such as natural grasses, bugs, or earthworms rather than grains. Standards are in flux and the food industry continues to lobby for a more lenient definition of what organic means. Hopefully, the organic industry will continue to tighten standards as they more closely monitor the classification and manufacturing of organic foods. Regardless of the organic industry's shortcomings, it's always best to choose organic whenever possible.

bacteria and our cells. Remember, bacteria are masters at effective communication—initiating it and interrupting it.

As you will learn, supporting our friendly bacteria with a comprehensive inside-out approach will help improve your health, enhance your energy, and heal from a wide range of illnesses including irritable bowel syndrome, ulcerative colitis, Crohn's disease, peptic ulcers, and even cancer and heart disease. But first, let's take a closer look at how we can better control the bad bugs.

Human Microbiome Project Update

An interview with Alan M Krensky, MD

To get an update on the Human Microbiome Project, we contacted Dr. Alan Krensky, former Deputy Director for the Office of Portfolio Analysis and Strategic Initiatives with the NIH. Authors Note: The next step in implementing the requirements of the NIH Health Reform Act of 2006, the NIH completed the organizational and administrative actions necessary to formally establish the Division of Program Coordination, Planning, and Strategic Initiatives (DPCPSI) within the Office of the Director. DPCPSI incorporates all of the functions of the existing Office of Portfolio Analysis and Strategic Initiatives (OPASI) as well as other program offices. With the dissolution of the OPASI, its former director, Dr. Alan Krensky, returned to his immunology lab at the National Cancer Institute to pursue his research interests full time. Dr. Lana Skirboll, director of the National Institutes of Health's Office of Science Policy, was named acting director of DPCPSI. Following is a portion of our interview with Dr. Krensky. For more information on the Human Microbiome Project refer to Chapter 7.

Q: What were the first steps to the Microbiome Project?

A: We jumpstarted the program in the Spring of 2007 with NIH funds. We felt it was important to start sequencing the microbes right away. We selected four sequencing centers that already had expertise in this area because of their work with the Human Genome Project. The goal of the centers was to sequence and list the various bacteria strains. In about six months, we already had 92 bacterial genomes sequenced. Within a year, we expect another 169. The target is 600, so we will be about one-third complete as a result of the jumpstart. We also created a data analysis and coordination center, which is a place to store the data that is collected. This means researchers have access to information about bacteria that was not available in the past.

The first phase also needs to establish consistent standards and deal with issues of informed consent documentation and other ethical matters. During this first phase, we also determined which sites we would test.

In men there are four sites and in women there are five—mouth, nose, GI [tract], skin, and vagina.

Q: How significant is it that this project analyzes bacteria from human volunteers?

A: It is very significant. By using human volunteers we can find out if there is a core microbial mix. We can determine if it changes seasonally or from one family member to another. We can determine if it changes after antibiotic use and, if so, how does it change. There are millions of questions to ask. By having human volunteers we can more accurately answer some of these questions. It will be done in a shotgun way just to get as much data in as possible. We will then piece it out to answer the many questions. The first steps are to have the repository and enhance our understanding of the sequencing of the multitude of microbes.

Q: What are the next steps?

A: After the jumpstart phase, we will award grants associated with the Microbiome Project to dozens of scientists in this area of study. In 2009, the grants total $28 million and are designed to look at the heart of the matter: How do microbes influence health and disease? We can find out from doctors and patients if there is a microbial pattern in illnesses such as chronic fatigue, depression, obesity, and other diseases. It's logical to assume that microbes are involved in diseases of the gut, but our hope is that we can go far beyond that, including mental health. If you recall, for years people with peptic ulcer disease were treated by psychiatrists before we found out that *H. pylori* bacteria was causing the disease. We may find out something similar with depression, schizophrenia, or other mental illnesses. Maybe we will find bacteria that play a significant role in diabetes or heart disease. There are huge, unthinkable things that can come from this work.

Q: When will we get some of these answers?

A: After the initial pilot phase, we will be able to quickly assess the projects to determine which ones should continue to get funding. We can expect some answers in the near future and shouldn't have to wait until the five-year term is complete. I think the pay-off of the project will be incredible.

3

MICROBIAL MONSTERS

THERE ARE TWO KEY WAYS that bacteria can negatively influence our health. A bad bacterium such as *E. coli*, *staph*, or *salmonella* can cause immediate gastrointestinal problems. Or an imbalance of bad to good bacteria can produce chronic, wide spread issues. (For information about specific harmful bacteria, refer to the chart on page 20.)

We've all heard the phrase, "Don't drink the water?" And many of us know what it feels like to have food that doesn't "agree with us." These are specific examples of *salmonella*, *E. coli*, or some other bacterial infiltration. There is a direct and isolated cause and effect—drink the water and get diarrhea or eat the food and get an upset stomach. But what happens when the bad bacteria are more insidious? What happens when the bacterial influence is not that clear cut? When bad bugs take over, the initial signs can be subtle and can eventually travel far beyond the gastrointestinal tract. Issues of bacterial imbalance can take months, even years, before they develop into a diagnosable disease. Let's take a closer look at what happens when bad bacteria cause chronic problems.

Systemic situation

The term systemic refers to our entire body system. When illnesses become systemic, they have moved beyond just one isolated part of the body and have become more widespread, influencing one or more body systems. As a result, they can also cause symptoms throughout the entire body. Rheumatoid arthritis, for example, can become a systemic illness when it affects other organs in addition to the joints. High blood pressure, diabetes, and cancer call all become systemic illnesses. The influenza virus is considered a systemic illness because it affects the entire body.

Rather than an isolated incidence, like eating bacteria-laced food that causes isolated symptoms like diarrhea, systemic bacterial battles are an ongoing power struggle between the good and the bad. Of course, in systemic cases, the bad bacteria have the upper hand. If the bad bacteria continually dominate, the end result can be serious illness.

There is a constant power struggle going on between good and bad bacteria. In most cases, the strongest bugs—good or bad—prevail. When the bad bugs are in control they can cause numerous initial symptoms. It's these symptoms that become the bacterial barometer of our internal ecosystem. It's important to notice the signs before your bacterial issues become systemic.

Signs to watch for

There is an old saying that we are sometimes unable to "see the forest for the trees." In other words, we can't see the big picture because we are so focused on the details. When it comes to health, the reverse is often true. We need to pay attention to each and every "tree." We are often only looking to prevent the "big illness." As a result, we sometimes miss the signs of an underlying illness that is percolating. To achieve and maintain optimal health, it's absolutely critical to get to know your body. Don't ignore signals that your body is sending you.

There are several preventive and diagnostic tests specific to the gastrointestinal tract. Some only need to be performed if there are specific symptoms and others should be done as a screening tool. These include:

- **Colonoscopy:** Used to view the large intestines; looking for inflamed tissue, abnormal growths (called polyps), and ulcers. This test is recommended every five years after the age of 50 or more frequently if there were any abnormalities like polyps previously found. If there is a family history of colon cancer, screening should begin at age 40.

- **Endoscopy:** Can detect abnormalities like inflammation or bleeding in the esophagus, stomach, and the first part of the small intestines that don't show up well on x-rays. This is done generally only if you have upper GI symptoms like GERD or ulcers.

- **Endoscopic Retrograde Cholangiopancreatography (ERCP):** A diagnostic test that can look at the liver, gallbladder, bile ducts, and pancreas.

- **Lower and Upper GI:** This x-ray looks at the lower GI (colon and rectum) and/or upper GI (esophagus, stomach, and part of the small intestine) and can detect abnormal growths, ulcers, polyps, or cancer.

- **Sigmoidoscopy:** A diagnostic tool that looks at the large intestines to find the cause of diarrhea, abdominal pain, or constipation. This test is rarely performed since the advent of the flexible colonoscopy.

- **Stool Analysis:** This test is done on feces to help diagnose infection from bacteria, viruses, or parasites.

- **Occult Blood Analysis:** This test is done on feces to look for blood. Often we may be bleeding from a diseased polyp but not know it because the blood is microscopic. This test helps find microscopic blood invisible to the naked eye. Occult blood analysis should be done at least yearly at your annual physical exam or by your gynecologist.

In addition to appropriate preventive care procedures, we need to take responsibility for recognizing our individual health signals. Our body, in its innate wisdom, sends us messages telling us how things are going. We need to listen to those messages. A thorough evaluation of signs and symptoms is one of the key ways that health issues associated with bacterial imbalance are diagnosed.

Here are ten key signals that our good bacteria are losing the battle:

- Bloating
- Gas
- Constipation
- Diarrhea
- Nausea
- Heartburn
- Food sensitivities
- Food cravings, specifically for sugar and refined carbohydrates
- Lack of energy
- Headaches or migraines

If you feel you may have a higher ratio of bad bacteria to good, ask yourself the questions featured on page 39. Your "yes" or "no" answers will give you the information you need. Chapters 4 and 11 provide detailed information about how you can shift that ratio.

Banning the bad guys

The idea of battling these bad bugs can seem overwhelming. However, there are simple things you can do to help reduce your exposure to harmful bacteria. It's impossible to avoid bad bacteria altogether, but we can certainly take proactive steps to limit our contact with unfriendly bacteria. Don't become too obsessive. Remember, interacting with bacteria can actually help strengthen your immune system. The following are some simple steps that you can take to reduce your exposure to harmful bacteria.

> *In order for a bacterial strain to be considered a probiotic, it must exert a clinically established health benefit.*

Let's start with the foods we eat. *Salmonella* and *E. coli* are the bacterial bad guys often found in foods. Some people can be carriers of these bacteria without showing overt symptoms of food poisoning. That's why it is critical that food handlers effectively wash their hands after using the restroom. The CDC reports that *salmonella* primarily originates in eggs, milk, poultry, and beef, however, there have also been outbreaks in peanut butter (remember that scare in 2008?) and unpasteurized fruit juice. Unfortunately, you can't tell if *salmonella* has contaminated food by smelling, tasting, or looking at it. Taking probiotics will help build up your resistance; however, we also must be diligent in how we choose and prepare foods. Wash your hands and food thoroughly, and rinse foods before cooking or eating, even if the food is in protective plastic wrapping.

Salmonella is not the only nasty bacterial strain that can infiltrate our food supply. *Escherichia coli* (E. coli) bacteria can cause food poisoning and is most famous for frequent recalls of hamburger. *E. coli* can also be found on fruits and vegetables.

According to an article in *The New York Times*, in 2000 and 2002 there were a record-setting 21 recalls of beef due to *E. coli* contamination, and in 2007, there were 20 recalls. In June 2008, the CDC reported that *salmonella* from tomatoes was blamed for an outbreak that caused fast-food giant McDonalds to temporarily remove all tomato slices from its sandwiches throughout the United States.

Helicobacter pylori (H. pylori) bacteria are also harmful microbes. *H. pylori* can be transmitted through human feces and municipal tap water. *H. pylori* have been found on a wide variety of foods including chicken and seafood.

Whether you work in the food supply/restaurant business or not, frequently and thoroughly washing hands is critical. Unfortunately, statistics show that many people do not wash their hands after using the restroom, and equally as many are not washing their hands properly. Here are some hand-washing tips to keep in mind:

- Use soap and warm water, and rinse thoroughly.
- Be sure to scrub between your fingers and get under your fingernails.
- Tightly press your palms together and be sure to wash the backs of your hands as well.
- The CDC recommend consistently washing your hands for a minimum of 20 seconds. If you don't have access to water, use a hand sanitizer product.
- Dry your hands using a clean towel.

In addition to washing after going to the bathroom, the CDC recommends you thoroughly wash your hands under the following circumstances:

- before and after preparing and eating food;
- after handling uncooked foods, particularly raw meat, poultry, or fish;
- before and after caring for someone who is sick;
- after blowing your nose, coughing, or sneezing; and
- after interacting with animals or handling animal waste.

Many studies have shown that children have fewer missed days of school due to gastrointestinal issues if they wash their hands properly. In addition, lower incidence of gastrointestinal problems in hospitals can directly be linked to proper hand washing of hospital staff. It's true, proper hand washing saves lives!

As for food, always be sure to maintain clean kitchen surfaces and use separate cutting boards for meats and vegetables. Be sure to thoroughly wash everything that touches raw meat. Chipped glasses and dishes should be thrown out because the cracks can harbor bad bacteria. Remember, bacteria can survive on surfaces for up to seven days. That's why routine cleaning of surfaces is important.

When it comes to tap water, we also need to be especially careful. As mentioned previously, a 2008 Associated Press investigation found many pharmaceuticals, including antibiotics, in municipal drinking water. In addition, there have been reports of a harmful strain of E. coli 0157:H7, in the drinking water of municipalities throughout the United States. A group of bacteria known as coliform are commonly found in drinking water. Some strains of E. coli, for example, are considered coliforms. In addition, a parasite found in water can cause the waterborne disease known as giardiasis. Numerous other chemicals such as lead, arsenic, and other toxins have been found in municipal drinking water.

To avoid bacteria, waterborne parasites, and toxins in the water you drink, avoid drinking municipal tap water. Drink pure bottled water or filtered water. Know the source of the water before drinking. Keep in mind that some bottled water companies actually use municipal water, so only drink brands from reputable bottlers that you trust.

Super-sized problem

Conventional wisdom has us paying meticulous attention to the bad bugs, but there is a debate as to the pros and cons of bacterial protection. No one would argue that we should stop washing our hands and our food. But have we gone too far when it comes to the battle we've waged against bacteria? According to a *Newsweek* expose provocatively titled *Caution: Killing Germs May Be Hazardous To Your Health*, we've gone way too far. It appears our super-sized sanitation efforts have led to super-sized problems. The authors tell us that new science is encouraging us to embrace bacteria.

"As antibiotics lose their effectiveness, researchers are returning to an idea that dates back to Pasteur, that the body's natural microbial flora aren't just an incidental fact of our biology, but crucial components of our health, intimate companions on an evolutionary journey that began millions of years ago," explains the *Newsweek* article.

In 1997, in response to our obsession with killing germs, McNeil Consumer Healthcare—makers of Tylenol, Benadryl, Visine, Bengay, and many other popular brands—introduced Purell hand sanitizer. They clearly had another hit on their hands. By capitalizing on people's germ phobia, McNeil managed to sell $90 million worth of Purell in 2006 alone. According to *Newsweek*, Purell and other alcohol gels have become a "part of the culture of cleanliness that's led to a different set of problems."

According to Dr. Levy, antibacterial cleansers are now a part of the problem because they can change the microbiology of the infectious agent. He told ABCNews.com that antibacterial cleansers should only be used by people who are seriously ill and especially vulnerable to bad bacteria or dangerous viruses. Even then, he says, they should be used on a limited basis.

Our germ-killing obsession has made us increasingly unable to fend off illnesses such as asthma, allergies, and autoimmune conditions (more about these conditions in Part Three). We've made a bad trade with the bugs. In exchange for the death of some bad bugs through extreme sanitation, we've weakened our immune systems, making us vulnerable to a whole host of other health issues. It appears as though our single focus on killing disease-causing germs has actually made them stronger.

So, do we just sit back and wait for the bad bugs to get us? Absolutely not. There are a number of factors that can help the good bacteria get stronger while keeping the bad bacteria at bay. The first course of action is to look at ways to stop antibiotic resistance.

Are You a Good Bacterial Best Friend?

To determine if your diet and lifestyle effectively supports your bacterial best friends, answer the following questions. If you answer yes to at least 75 percent of these questions, you win the Bacterial Best Friend of the Year award. If you have more no answers than yes, you are letting down your bacterial buddies and you need to work on being a better friend.

Diet	yes	no
I drink about eight 8-ounce cups of water each day.		
I limit my alcohol to no more than one drink per day.		
I eat at least three servings of vegetables every day.		
I eat at least two servings of fruits every day.		
I eat whole grains instead of processed flour products.		
I do not eat red meat more than three times per week.		
I eat fresh fish at least twice a week.		
I eat organic food as much as possible to avoid preservatives, additives, hormones, antibiotics, and other toxins.		
I avoid trans fats and choose monounsaturated fats such as olive and macadamia nut oils.		
I limit my intake of refined carbohydrates and simple sugars.		
I do not eat at fast food restaurants.		
I eat 25 grams of fiber each day.		
Lifestyle		
I exercise for 30 minutes at least four times a week.		
I employ effective stress relieving techniques.		
I get seven to eight hours of sleep at least five nights a week.		
I would say that I am generally a very happy person.		
I have loving and supportive people in my life.		

Stopping antibiotic resistance

We certainly don't want to go back to the days of infectious disease pandemics and unsanitary conditions. But there are steps that must be taken if we are to stop the dangerous trend of antibiotic resistance. At this rate, if we don't reduce antibiotic resistance, the bad bugs will continue to dominate us.

If we really want to ease antibiotic resistance, we need to do three things:

- Stop over prescribing and misusing antibiotic drugs.
- Employ a diet and lifestyle that strengthens our own defenses while inhibiting the growth of bad bacteria rather than enhancing their power.
- Stop feeding antibiotics to our livestock and poultry unless it is absolutely medically necessary.

"While the most direct cause of antibiotic resistance is prescription use," explains Sachs, "evidence continues to grow that resistant bacteria and their dangerous genes are reaching us via the meat, eggs, and polluted runoff coming out of livestock operations."

It is critical that the United States and Canada follow the example set by the European Union (representing 27 member states in Europe) on January 1, 2006. According to the Union of Concerned Scientists (www.ucsusa.org), the European Union banned feeding of all antibiotics and related drugs to livestock for growth promotion purposes.

"In the United States, antibiotics and related drugs are used routinely to encourage growth and to compensate for crowded and unsanitary conditions in the production of poultry, swine, and cattle," reports the Union of Concerned Scientists. According to the Organic Consumers Association, three million pounds of antibiotics are administered to Americans each year, while nearly 25 million pounds of antibiotics are administered to livestock for purposes other than treating disease.

Although North America has not yet banned the use of antibiotics as the European Union has, there is a robust organic foods movement. In 2003, North America actually exceeded Europe for the first time as the largest market for organic food and drink. To avoid antibiotics in foods, buy organic meat, eggs, poultry, and dairy (for more information about organics refer to the side bar on page 41).

CHAPTER

4

FRIENDS FOREVER

THE TERM FRIENDSHIP CAN MEAN different things to different people. Typically, however, when we think of a friend, we think of someone we can rely on, confide in, and trust. A friend is loyal and committed, quickly at your side during times of need. A friend helps you celebrate your victories, shares in your joy, and comforts you when you are in pain.

Perhaps Ralph Waldo Emerson said it best: "A friend may well be reckoned the masterpiece of nature." And nature provides us with many unique opportunities for friendship. Whether your best friend has four legs and you found him at the pound, or is your sister that you have known for decades, friendship is a gift. As the famous Greek philosopher Aristotle said, "Friendship is a single soul dwelling in two bodies."

As we take a closer look at bacteria, could it be that we have billions of "friends" dwelling in one body? We think so.

Making friends

So far, we've talked a lot about bad bacteria. But it's time to get to know the billions of friendly bacteria that inhabit our internal ecosystem. After all, as Abraham Lincoln once said, "The best way to destroy an enemy is to make a friend." And the more friendly bacteria we have, the less likelihood that our enemies will be able to enter. But what exactly are friendly bacteria? As mentioned previously, our bacterial best friends are called probiotics, a.k.a. "good bacteria."

Probiotics are living microorganisms that are similar to the beneficial bacteria found in the human gut. As we have evolved over millions of years, we have developed a complex and symbiotic relationship with the trillions of microscopic organisms living in and on us. New science is showing us that there is a microbial element to every aspect of our health.

Probiotics are found in foods and dietary supplements. Gregor Reid, PhD, professor of microbiology at the University of Western Ontario, Canada, explains that a big misconception is that probiotics are inside us. "They are not inside us unless we ate some," he says. Probiotics are meant to strengthen and feed the good bacteria we were born with. In order for the good bacteria to outnumber the bad, we need to replenish them by eating probiotics.

Friendly bacteria are created through a process of fermentation. Fermentation is used to create many common foods including vinegar, olives, cheese, yogurt, and bread. This biochemical process occurs when a microorganism breaks down substances into smaller pieces.

A long time ago, the fermentation of vegetables was perfected by Asian cultures. One popular and well-known fermented Asian food is miso. Miso is created by grinding soybeans into a paste. Tempeh is also a fermented soy probiotic product. Tempeh uses the whole soybean to create a cake form. Here in the United States, tempeh is thought of as a "health food," but in Malaysia, it is considered a delicacy. Many epidemiological studies have shown that the Asian diet, which is high in miso and tempeh, provides many health benefits. In Chapter 7 we will feature an in-depth interview with award-winning microbiologist Iichiroh Ohhira, PhD, who has combined the ancient

Want to lose weight? Ask your friends for some help!

Are you gaining weight? New research says you can blame it on the bugs. Bacteria can do many things. Bad bacteria can make us sick and friendly bacteria can make us well. But can bacteria really make us fat or thin? Researchers from Washington University found that there is a direct link between bacteria and weight loss. In early 2008, Jeffrey Gordon, MD, and his research team found that as obese individuals lost weight, there was an increase in one particular strain of gut bacteria. Gordon had previously demonstrated that bacteria affects the body's ability to extract calories from food and regulate genes involved in energy metabolism, two key issues associated with weight loss or gain.

Researchers from the University of Calgary demonstrated that prebiotics can also help individuals lose weight. Their study featuring 48 overweight and obese adults received 21 grams of prebiotics versus a placebo (fake pill) for 12 weeks. At the end of the study, people taking the prebiotic lost an average of 2.3 pounds while the people taking the fake pill actually gained an average of 1 pound. The researchers speculate that daily consumption of a prebiotic may be able to suppress levels of hormones linked to hunger. The study, which was published in the June 2009 issue of the *American Journal of Clinical Nutrition*, also demonstrated an improvement in glucose regulation in the people taking the prebiotic.

According to a *Newsweek* magazine article, the genetic factors associated with weight control may reside in the genes of our bacteria. "Regrettably, it turns out that bacteria exhibit a strong preference for making us fat," conclude the *Newsweek* authors. New research, however, demonstrates the importance of supporting our "good" bacteria. According to the president of the World Gastrointerology Association, Eamonn Quigley, MD, combating obesity is proving to be a significant and exciting new application for probiotics.

The lesson? If you are engaged in the battle of the bulge, you need to get the right bugs on your side. To lose weight, repopulate, support, and strengthen your friendly bacteria with probiotics. Probiotics, combined with a healthy diet and exercise, may help you achieve your weight loss goals.

We'll address the issue of probiotics and weight loss in more detail in Part Three.

art of Japanese fermentation with modern science to create a potent probiotic known as Dr. Ohhira's Probiotics 12 PLUS.

According to the World Health Organization, if probiotics are ingested in adequate amounts, they can provide a variety of health benefits to humans. The expanding science regarding the benefits of probiotics has lead to a dramatic increase in probiotic foods and supplements.

The National Center for Complementary and Alternative Medicine (NCCAM) reports that sales of probiotic supplements in the United States nearly tripled from 1994 to 2003. This topic is so interesting that the NCCAM, in connection with the American Society for Microbiology, held a conference in November 2005 to explore the use of probiotics for the prevention and treatment of a variety of health conditions. The conference found encouraging evidence for the use of probiotics for:

- diarrhea, especially in infants;
- urinary and female genital tract infections;
- irritable bowel syndrome;
- bladder cancer prevention;
- intestinal infections caused by *Clostridium difficile*;
- pouchitis (acute inflammation that can occur after colon removal); and
- eczema in children.

NCCAM-sponsored research involving probiotics is presently taking place at Tulane University, Mayo Clinic College of Medicine, and Tufts-New England Medical Center.

In Part Three, we will go into much more detail about the various conditions that can benefit from probiotics. You don't have to have a specific illness, however, to glean the benefits from friendly bacteria. If you are pro-health, you need probiotics. In fact, ingesting probiotics and supporting friendly bacteria are the essential missing links to optimal health and vitality for everyone, not just those stricken with a serious illness.

Flaxseed Tips

Flax oil has become a popular dietary supplement. It is not a cooking oil but it can be put on salads, in oatmeal, or simply taken by the tablespoon. Flaxseed oil must be refrigerated and it will only last for about two months. Never take flaxseed oil if it is not fresh. If you have some flax oil that is older than two months, try using it on your wood cabinets. We have found that it makes a perfect polish.

If the taste of pure flaxseed oil is not appealing, you can get the same health benefits by grinding flaxseeds in your coffee grinder. You can then sprinkle the seeds on oatmeal, salads, yogurt, and other healthful foods. Do not over-grind the seeds because the increased heat can break down the fatty acid content, thereby reducing the health benefits.

How probiotics help us

It's interesting that probiotic means "for life" while antibiotic means "against life." We know that probiotics are antimicrobial because they release bacteriocins that actually kill bad bacteria. But what else can our billion best friends do for us. We've described in detail what happens when the bad bacteria take over, so now let's look at what happens when the good guys win.

Without bacteria the Earth would look like the moon—devoid of life, water, wind, and even air. The good bacteria in our bodies serve many critical functions that can be placed in four important categories:

- Immune system
- Digestion
- Detoxification and elimination
- Cellular activity

Let's take a closer look at each of these, beginning with the immune system.

Many of us only think of our immune system when we get sick. It's top of mind when we have the flu, for example. But most days we forget that we even have such an incredible internal defense system. The immune system is a mysterious matrix of cells, tissues, and organs designed to keep us healthy.

"Living on a planet teeming with hungry microorganisms and coated with protein and sugar, the human body is a feast to microscopic life—and the only thing standing between 'us' and 'them' is the immune system," writes Robert Roundtree, MD, and Carol Colman in their book, *Immunotics*.

The immune system is made up of trillions of specialized cells with one common goal: keep the host (that's us) healthy. Learning about the immune system is like curling up with a juicy novel. There is suspense, loyalty, and the thrill of the chase as our immune system cells hunt down foreign invaders. Even the names of some of the immune system players are dramatic: macrophages, leukocytes, and natural killer cells. And then there is the softer side of the immune system with T-cells, B-cells, and helper cells. Together they all make up a first-rate team working on our behalf.

We think you'll be surprised as to where most of these amazing immune system cells reside in the body. About 70 percent of the immune system is located in and around the gut. That's right, the same place where bacteria like to call home. If we want a strong immune system, we need to support the friendly bacteria living along side our immune system cells in the gut.

In addition to the immune system, good bacteria play a vital role in digestion. Your digestive system has constant contact with our outside world, so it makes sense that it would be exposed to bad bugs on a consistent basis. Methodically, the digestive system turns food into fuel. After we eat, the digestive system breaks down the food, tests for microbes, extracts nutrients, and eliminates the excess. This system is easily taken for granted when everything is running smoothly.

Healthy Fiber Alternatives

When things aren't running smoothly, it may be tempting to reach for the most popular drug-store brand of fiber to add to your daily diet. Adding fiber to the diet may be a great idea, but it's really important to choose the right fiber. You may be surprised to find out that the most well-known fiber powder supplement contains 9 grams of sugar. The capsules contain four different toxic preservatives including polysorbate 80 and several artificial colorings. Why does a capsule even need artificial colorings in the first place? And don't choose the wafers either. With this same brand, two of the wafers have just as much sugar as they do fiber. Even the manufacturer warns that the wafers should not be used by people who are diabetic or on a calorie-restricted diet.

What do we do when we are not running like a well-oiled machine? Choose foods high in fiber or dietary fiber supplements that do not contain artificial ingredients and high amounts of sugar. Here are our high fiber food choices:

- **First choice:** Legumes like lentils, black beans, and chick peas have between 13 to 15 grams of fiber per one cup.

- **Second choice:** Vegetables like green beans, spinach, and broccoli offer anywhere from 4 to 5 grams per one cup serving.

- **Third choice:** Whole grains like bran cereal and whole wheat bread. (Tip: Choose whole wheat whenever possible. One cup of whole-wheat spaghetti delivers 6 grams of fiber compared to about 1 gram for standard pasta.)

It's important to add more fiber to the diet, but be sure it's the right type of fiber.

However, if something is amiss with digestion, you will most likely notice it right away.

At some point, most of us have experienced times when digestion does not go smoothly—gas, bloating, heartburn, etc. Good bacteria help us avoid the discomforts and illnesses associated with poor digestion. Equally important, our bacterial buddies also help us prevent leaky gut syndrome (we'll address this important aspect of digestion in more detail in Part Three).

Friendly bacteria not only help us digest foods, they also help support efficient detoxification and elimination. When foods are not eliminated properly we get constipated. It's not good to have toxic waste sitting in our bodies for too long. It's important to have a well-formed, easy-to-pass bowel movement at least once a day. Our friendly bacteria help us filter out toxins and disable pathogens so they can be effectively eliminated. Efficient detoxification and elimination is absolutely critical to optimum health.

Good bacteria also support proper cellular activity on a variety of levels. Good bacteria produce important vitamins such as vitamin K and biotin. Without vitamin K, we could bleed to death because our blood would not clot. Vitamin K is also critical to bone health. Biotin serves many important roles in the body with its primary function being the metabolism of fats, proteins, and carbohydrates. New preliminary unpublished research shows that beneficial bacteria can even promote satiety, that feeling of being full and satisfied. "Initial results in a previous research project indicate that specific probiotic derivatives do have an interesting satiety effect," explained Arne Astrup, MD, PhD, of the University of Copenhagen. Perhaps producing biotin and encouraging satiety is how probiotics help with weight loss; however, more study in this area is needed before we can draw definitive conclusions regarding weight loss.

As you can see, there is a long list of reasons why we should support the billion best friends living in our bodies. We can do this through diet, lifestyle, and probiotic supplements.

Sugar and fat

"Bacteria keep us alive," explains Dr. Reid, "yet our food system severely lacks restoring and enhancing them." That's because the American diet is woefully lacking in vital nutrients.

It's fitting that the acronym for the standard American diet is SAD. The corner stone of this SAD diet is sugar. Not simply sugar directly sprinkled on food from a sugar bowl, but high fructose corn syrup hidden in many foods. Ketchup, peanut butter, some crackers, and even the probiotic-friendly food yogurt can have lots of added sugar. The worst culprits are soft drinks. Just one 12-ounce can of soda contains about 40 grams of sugar—that's ten teaspoons.

According to a 2005 WebMD report, on average Americans consume about 13 pounds of added sugar every month. Such excesses of sugar directly cause obesity, and will also feed bad bacteria and weaken good bacteria.

Even healthful foods contain too much sugar. One of the most commonly purchased brands of yogurt has 17 grams of sugar in just one four-ounce serving. There's even sugar hiding in other "health foods" like fiber. The most popular powdered fiber supplement sold in pharmacies has a whopping 9 grams of sugar in just one tablespoon. For more information on healthy fiber alternatives, refer to page 63. Chapter 11 goes into more detail about the dangers of sugar.

High fat is another common characteristic of the standard American diet. A person who is not very active and consuming a 2,000-calorie diet should not eat more than 60 grams of fat per day. To put that into perspective, if you have a Big Mac, French fries, and a milk shake for lunch, you are already over your fat intake limit for the entire day.

But not all fats are bad. There are good fats that should be in the diet. These fats are called essential fatty acids (EFAs). We'll discuss EFAs in more detail in Chapter 11 but here is a quick overview. Fat is one of the most misunderstood foods available. Just as there are good bacteria and bad bacteria, there are good fats and bad fats. Essential fatty acids (EFAs) are the good fats. Omega-3 and omega-6 are the two main categories of essential fatty acids.

Most saturated fats are found in animal products like butter, cheese, whole milk, cream, and fatty meats.

Trans fats are deadly and are added to a wide variety of products to enhance shelf life. These dangerous fats are also used in many restaurants. Because of the damaging health effects of trans fats, in January 2006, the Federal Food and Drug Administration required food manufacturers to list both saturated and trans fat amounts on the label. Because trans fats have been directly linked to cancer, heart disease, and many other illnesses, some major cities throughout the United States have banned their use in restaurants.

Monounsaturated and polyunsaturated fats are considered good fats. Polyunsaturated fats must have a balance of 1:1 of omega-3 and omega-6 essential fatty acids. Some fats are meant to be taken as dietary supplements and some are meant to be cooked with. Fats that should never be heated and only taken as dietary supplements include:

- Flaxseed oil
- Fish oil
- Borage oil
- Evening primrose oil
- Hemp seed oil
- Black currant oil

An ideal oil to cook with is Australian premium macadamia nut oil. This oil contains the highest amount of monounsaturated fats—the healthiest kind of fat—and is extremely stable. One of the reasons we recommend this oil for cooking is because it can be used at very high temperatures including searing, browning, deep-frying, and high-temperature baking. We recommend MacNut Oil because of the effective processing and packaging that helps maintain the other naturally-occurring nutrients such as vitamin E, carotenes, and phospholipids.

Made famous by the Mediterranean Diet, one of the most common "healthy" oils for cooking is olive oil. Keep in mind, however, that the cooking temperature for this oil should not exceed 320 degrees. This makes olive oil appropriate for light sautéing, low-heat baking, and pressure cooking. The more refined the oil, the more it has been subjected to process and the less healthy it is—which is why extra-virgin olive oil is the healthiest type of olive oil. Please note, there is a lengthy discussion of oils and fats in Dr. Pescatore's best-selling book, *The Hamptons Diet* (Wiley 2004).

To maintain the proper balance of essential fatty acids, avoid oils high in omega-6s including corn, safflower, sunflower, soybean, or cottonseed. We recommend taking a high quality omega-3 supplement every day. Many people take a fish oil dietary supplement because fish oils have been clearly demonstrated to help prevent heart disease and cancer. Dr. Ohhira's Essential Living Oils is a vegetarian alternative to fish oils. The Dr. Ohhira product is exclusively distributed by Essential Formulas and contains eight different essential plant oils.

In addition to fish oils, flaxseed oil is often taken as a dietary supplement. Flaxseed oil is the highest plant-based source of omega-3 fatty acids. It should never be used for cooking. For more information on flax, refer to the side bar on page 61.

Support strategy overview

The top two things you can do to help strengthen your bacterial best friends are to reduce your sugar intake and eliminate bad fats while increasing your consumption of good fats. Here are some other critical dietary strategies that will help you tip the bacterial scales in favor of the friendly:

- **Eat more fruits and vegetables.** Many fruits and vegetables are considered "prebiotic" and will help support probiotics (more about prebiotics in Part II).
- **Avoid processed and preserved food.** These foods feed the bad bacteria and leave the good bacteria feeling hungry.
- **Eat probiotic foods.** Probiotic foods contain health-promoting live bacteria and include yogurt (without sugar, preservatives, and additives), kefir, miso, and tempeh.

- **Eat enough fiber.** Between 25 and 30 grams of fiber is required to encourage healthy digestion and elimination.
- **Rotate your diet based on the change of seasons.** This will encourage you to eat fresh, seasonal foods.
- **Eat more fish.** Cold-water fish have important omega-3 fatty acids such as EPA and DHA that support proper bacterial balance.
- **Drink plenty of pure water.** Water helps flush out toxins, encourages proper elimination, and hydrates the cells.

To determine if you are properly supporting your good bacteria, take the test on page 53.

In addition to what you eat and drink, what you *do* can help support your internal bacterial best friends. Your actions send messages to your friendly bacteria and we certainly don't want to send them the wrong message.

Our good bacteria hate stress just as much as we do. Conversely, bad bacteria just love it when we are under stress because it helps them grow. Practicing stress reduction techniques will go a long way toward helping to support your good bacteria. In today's world, it is nearly impossible to rid our daily lives of stress. And let's face it, some stress is good—your wedding, a promotion, or even your relationships with loved ones. The issue is not to eliminate stress completely but to discover effective stress relief techniques that work for you. This is such an important topic we'll go over it in detail in Chapter 11.

Exercise is a great stress-relieving technique. But exercise does a lot more than reduce stress. Numerous studies have shown that exercise strengthens the immune system, builds strong bones and muscles, reduces obesity, enhances mental function, improves emotional well-being, and positively influences nearly every key system in the human body. It's no wonder that consistent exercise can contribute to a healthy bacterial balance as well.

Exercise is critical to our good health but let's face it, it's hard to exercise if we are tired. That's why sleep is really the unsung hero of health-promotion. In today's fast-paced world, many of us are sleep deprived. We often wear that fact like a badge of honor, not realizing the serious damage that lack of sleep can cause. Exciting research from the Sleep and Neuroimaging Lab at the University of California, Berkeley, is confirming the broad health impacts of sleep. Lead researcher Matthew Walker, PhD, says sleep is just as important to our survival as food. Dr. Walker says that studies have proven that animals will die just as quickly from sleep deprivation as from food deprivation. Dr. Walker and his research team are showing that lack of sleep can cause significant impairment of the immune system and brain function, even leading to symptoms associated with psychological disorders. We are sure that controlled research in the future will show us exactly how lack of sleep impairs proper bacterial balance. If you want your bacterial best friends to be healthy, be sure they get a good night's sleep—seven to eight hours every night.

It's not surprising that the same things that keep us healthy also keep our good bacteria healthy and thriving. Our comprehensive inside-out ultimate health plan is featured in detail in Chapter 11.

Most Americans do not have the proper balance of good bacteria to bad. In fact, many have the opposite ratio of far more bad than good. It is the imbalance of bad to good bacteria that may be linked to nearly every serious illness known. In addition, even marginal deficiencies of good bacteria can cause uncomfortable symptoms and disrupt the quality of life. If we are to thrive, not just survive, we need to help our good bacteria do the same.

PART TWO
REPOPULATE PROPERLY

CHAPTER

5

PROBIOTIC PALS

THERE ARE A VARIETY OF ways we can achieve optimum health. We can exercise, eat a nutritious diet, practice stress management, get enough sleep, and focus on a healthy lifestyle. Even if we do all of that, we may continue to struggle if we do not have a healthy internal bacterial balance. Most health concerns can be linked, at least in part, to bacterial imbalance. If we are to have active, vibrant lives, we need to support the body at its core. Probiotics provide the bacterial bedrock we need to be healthy. We are convinced that understanding the role of healthy bacterial balance is a critical missing link to optimum health.

Author and oncologist Jeremy Geffen, MD, refers to the human body as a "precious and wondrously complex garden—rather than a machine." When talking about bacteria, we really like this wonderful analogy of the body as a garden. When it comes to your "inner garden," you can and should replant the seeds of good bacteria that are constantly being depleted. When gardening, there is sometimes the temptation to only focus on the weeds—or in the case of our health, the symptoms. But by focusing on enhancing our friendly bacteria, we can create a lush inner garden that leads to vibrant health with far fewer "weeds."

For the past 100 years, the mainstream medical community has viewed all bacteria as bad. As we mentioned in Part One, we've blasted the bad bugs with antibiotics and scrubbed them with antimicrobial agents, only to find that we have actually made them stronger. In many cases, the weeds in the garden have taken over. But it's time to take a closer look at the garden we have created and find ways to enhance its growing power. It's time to shift our focus from our bacterial enemies to our probiotic pals.

Probiotics are the antithesis of harmful bacteria. After all, that's why they are referred to as "good bacteria." For everything negative that harmful bacteria can do, probiotics can do the opposite. Probiotics can help strengthen the immune system, reduce chronic inflammation, and help prevent and treat leaky gut syndrome. Through a process of fermentation, lactic acid bacteria are produced to create effective probiotics, which are found in some foods and available as dietary supplements. This chapter will take an in-depth look at how we can properly repopulate our probiotic pals.

There are friendly bacteria we are born with and ones that are just passing through. Both are valuable. One person may have a strain of bacteria firmly adhered to his colon wall, while that same bacteria is transient in another person. But if we are to achieve the 85 percent to 15 percent good to bad ratio, we need to find ways to support the good bacterial strains we were born with, even if we don't know exactly what those strains are. One of the ways we do this is by choosing the most effective, viable, and comprehensive probiotic possible.

Remember, however, that bad bacteria are stubborn and tough. Simply adding in good bacteria is not enough. We need to make sure we use a probiotic product that is potent enough to actually kill the bad bacteria while repopulating the good.

Who needs probiotics?

We are often asked if probiotics are even necessary. The simple answer is that, as long as you are alive, you need probiotics. The

Do you need probiotics?

If you are wondering if you should take a probiotic supplement, take this simple quiz.

	yes	no
Have you been on an antibiotic within the past year?		
Are you under stress that interrupts the quality of your life?		
Do you eat poorly several times a week?		
Do you have a sedentary lifestyle with very little physical activity?		
Have you been diagnosed with a serious illness within the past 12 months?		
Have you experienced diarrhea or constipation within the past three months?		
Have you had a urinary tract infection within the past three months?		
Do you have food allergies, outdoor allergies, or asthma?		
Do you have acne, eczema or other skin problems?		
Do you ever experience heartburn, gas, or bloating after you eat?		
Do you frequently get colds and flu?		
Do you travel frequently?		
Are you overweight by at least 10 pounds?		
Do you have a family history of cancer, heart disease, or diabetes?		
Total		

If you answered yes, to at least half of the questions, you definitely need a probiotic.

only variable is to what degree. One person may show no signs of bacterial imbalance and will only take probiotics for a few weeks out of the entire year. A few people may even be able to get all the good bacteria they need from food. While others may need to take a probiotic every day, similar to their multi-vitamin/mineral supplement. Certainly if individuals are experiencing a specific health issue, probiotics are a critical addition to their health-promoting strategy. In Chapter 10, we have described all of the major conditions that can be related to bacterial balance. These conditions will be helped tremendously by probiotics.

If you have an ideal balance of bacteria, you may not need to take probiotics very often or at all. However, given the stresses of our daily existence and the toxic environments in which we live, we think it is safe to assume that everyone will need a daily probiotic. How do you know if you have enough friendly bacteria? It's simple, if you are experiencing certain symptoms, you don't have enough good bacteria. Bad bacteria cause digestive disturbances such as gas, bloating, constipation, diarrhea, and others, as well as issues with the skin,

Probiotics For Kids

Many studies have clearly demonstrated that probiotics can help ease diarrhea in children after onset. But what about prevention? Do probiotics help protect kids against bacterial and viral infections? According to a 2009 study featured in the journal *Vaccine*, a probiotic supplement reduced viral infections by 18 percent. There was also a significant reduction observed regarding bacterial infections and gastrointestinal disease.

Probiotics are safe for children at any age. If a child has been on an antibiotic, it is especially recommended that supplemental probiotics be used to help re-establish proper bacterial balance. Taken daily, probiotics can help a child have a strong digestive system and immune function.

continual colds and flu, poor energy, and numerous other symptoms, any of which can indicate you have more bad than good bacteria. You can take the quiz on page 75 to see where you stand.

Whether you are having symptoms of bacterial imbalance or not, taking probiotics during and after antibiotic use is absolutely critical. It's best to take the probiotic at a different time than the antibiotic. You should also continue to take a high-quality probiotic twice a day for at least two weeks after you stop taking your antibiotic.

Although people with a perfect bacterial balance are virtually non-existent due to our high stress lifestyles and poor food quality, there are certain populations who are especially in need of probiotic supplements including:

- People with digestion and elimination issues.
- Women who are pregnant.
- Infants born via cesarean section.
- Infants who are not being breast-fed.
- Children and adults who have been on antibiotics.
- Anyone previously diagnosed with or suffering from a serious illness.
- The elderly.
- People eating a poor diet or those who are inactive.
- Individuals experiencing unusually high amounts of stress and anxiety.
- People taking prescription or over-the-counter drugs on a regular basis.

By properly populating the friendly bacteria, we increase the probability that those bacteria will stick to the colon wall so there is less room for harmful bacteria to take up residence. It was previously thought that all we had to do to restore bacterial balance was to inundate the colon with friendly bacteria—the more, the better. This concept, which emphasizes the number of colony forming units (CFUs), is definitely outdated.

The numbers game

The way we have been using probiotics is similar to how we use (or should we say misuse) antibiotics. The theory is that we need more antibiotics to kill all the bad bugs. We have clearly shown the error in that thinking. However, we have been applying that same basic principle to our probiotic supplements—more is better. But that's not the case.

Just as we have tried to blast out the bugs with antibiotics, we are now trying to overpower them with large quantities of the friendly folks. For years, consumers have been told to read the label carefully and look for the number of organisms—the bigger the number the better. To some degree, that makes perfect sense. If probiotics are good for us why wouldn't more be better? However, it's just not that simple.

"Our research demonstrated that simply flooding the body with microflora did not lead to good health," explains award-winning Japanese researcher Iichiroh Ohhira, PhD. "The consumption of high CFU probiotics encourages the body to sense that the flora are 'foe' rather than 'friend' and can activate the body's defense mechanisms."

The immune system is already set up to instantaneously determine if a new cell is an enemy invader or an ally. If the immune cells are overwhelmed by what they perceive as invading bad bacteria, they will react and activate T and B cells. Sometimes an overactive immune system can be just as dangerous as an under-active one. An overactive immune system can lead to serious autoimmune conditions such as rheumatoid arthritis, lupus, or multiple sclerosis. For years, Dr. Ohhira has been focused on the quality and viability of the bacteria versus the quantity. For more information about Dr. Ohhira's philosophy and research findings, refer to page 98.

When a manufacturer refers to their product as having a "higher potency" they are only referring to the number of CFUs. This is misleading. Potency does not mean quantity, it means strength and effectiveness. A high CFU product may, in fact, not be potent at all.

Two most common bacterial species

Lactobacillus and *bifidobacterium* are the two most common species of bacteria. *Lactobacillus acidophilus* has become so mainstream that many people refer to their probiotic supplement as merely "acidophilus." The *bifidobacterium* is so important to the colon that one manufacturer has invented the term "bifidus regularis," trying to convey to consumers that their yogurt will help keep them "regular." As an aside, in January 2008, that same manufacturer was sued in Los Angels Federal Court for making false and misleading claims about the health benefits of bifidus regularis. At the time this book was published, that lawsuit has not yet been resolved.

Bifidobacterium are one of the key species of bacteria that live in the colon. The most well-known *Bifidobacterium* strain is *Bifidobacterium longum*, however several other strains such as *Bifidobacterium breve* and *Bifidobacterium infantis* are also beneficial.

Lactobacillus acidophilus primarily live in the intestines and the vagina. In addition to acidophilus, there are several *lactobacillus* strains that have demonstrated effectiveness including *Lactobacillus brevis*, *Lactobacillus bulgaricus*, and *Lactobacillus casei*.

When taking a probiotic supplement, be sure it contains several of the *bifidobacterium* and *lactobacillus* strains.

Some of the "high potency" products on the market contain a high number of CFUs "at the time of manufacture." Those bacteria may not be viable when they finally reach your intestines. That's the reason manufacturers focus so intently on enormous CFU numbers. If they are not sure the bacteria will survive long enough to make it to your gut, they simply add more bacteria so they have a better chance of getting more bacteria to stick. This practice is not an exact science. If a manufacturer is confident that their bacteria will survive, they will not focus as much on a high CFU number. The survivability of the bacteria once they are inside the human body is the most critical aspect of an effective probiotic.

Be aware that cultured dairy-based probiotics—yogurt in particular—are notorious for having a very low percentage survival rate of the good bacteria. Also it's worth repeating that if you are going to rely on yogurt as your primary probiotic source (and that's certainly a strategy we would never recommend), be sure to choose an organic yogurt brand that does not contain added sugar.

The final word on CFUs is that if the bacteria are dead when they get to your gut, CFUs are a non-issue. Even if there are *trillions* of bacteria in the probiotic, if the bacteria are not viable when they reach the intestines, the product is useless. Dosages vary based on individual circumstances and health status.

If the bacteria are viable, CFUs are important—but it is just one factor. It is also critical to know exactly which strains we are ingesting. There is much debate as to which of the different strains of lactic acid bacteria are the most effective. Most studies have followed the pharmaceutical standard of research by studying just one strain, such as the *lactobacillus* or *bifidobacterium* species. Several studies have been done using the *lactobacillus rhamnosus* GG strain. While these

Probiotic Safety

There is no recommended daily allowance (RDA) for probiotics. Probiotic supplements are generally considered safe. The most common side effect, oddly enough, could be GI discomfort. Women who are nursing, pregnant, or planning on becoming pregnant should discuss taking a probiotic with their physician. Individuals taking prescription medications should also consult with their physician before taking any nutritional supplement. Having said that, unfortunately many physicians have not even heard of probiotics and, if they have, they are not well versed in choosing an effective probiotic supplement, so you are left to use your own better judgment.

Mother's Milk

There have been many studies demonstrating that babies who are breast-fed are healthier. New research shows that one of the reasons this may be the case is because human breast milk contains more than 130 different combinations of oligosaccharides, which are foods that help good bacteria fight harmful organisms. These important prebiotics also help enhance the strength of the good bacteria the baby is born with.

studies have been successful, keep in mind that there are more than 100 different *lactobacillus* species.

It was previously thought that the *lactobacillis acidophilus (L. acidophilus)* species was the most significant strain, making "acidophilus" a household term. Other strains of *lactobacillus* are proving to be more important than *L. acidophilus*. We should not focus all of our attention on just one strain. There are more than 400 different species of bacteria living in the human gut, each having hundreds of different strains. Dr. Ohhira found that flooding the system with just one or two strains does not appear to be the answer.

Although using a variety of different strains is important, it's even more important that the friendly bacteria thrive once inside. Bacterial viability after ingestion is the most important aspect concerning probiotics.

In order for a probiotic to be viable, it must address issues that go beyond total CFUs including:

- incorporating many complementary strains versus just one or two isolated strains;
- delivering prebiotics that help feed probiotic bacteria;
- providing enzyme activity to aid digestion, reduce inflammation, and alleviate toxins; and
- helping to normalize pH balance in the colon.

Using the most effective probiotic supplement will help recondition the pH of the colon. This will not only kill harmful bacteria, it will also provide an environment conducive for the growth of friendly bacteria. To help us stay healthy, the colon must maintain optimum pH, which is the acid to alkaline balance. Friendly bacteria thrive in a balanced pH environment while harmful bacteria prefer a higher acid-to-alkaline ratio. When a probiotic supplement helps normalize pH, it is also supporting the good bacterial strains you were born with.

In addition to enzyme activity and normalizing pH, we need quality and synergy. The end result isn't just a pill filled with good bacteria.

Probiotics plus

How do we make something good even better? We find things that complement it and we combine them. Take a moment to think of a great relationship between two people. Both people are wonderful, unique individuals, but when they come together they enhance each other and create a complementary union of strengths, skills, emotions, and a rhythmic happiness. The same is true for our probiotic pals. Alone they are amazing microbes, but when combined with prebiotics, they form a marriage made in heaven.

Prebiotics are non-digestible food fibers that help stimulate the growth and activity of specific, friendly bacterial strains. When you combine probiotics with prebiotics it is known as a synbiotic. Synbiotics are effective at lower dosages because the prebiotic enhances the effectiveness of the probiotic. As we've previously reported, many studies have shown that prebiotics alone have their own health-promoting properties.

After years of meticulous research, Dr. Ohhira has developed an innovative fermentation process that helps create naturally-occurring prebiotics. The synbiotic created by Dr. Ohhira is produced using a three-year natural temperature fermentation process. He

Are soil-based organisms safe?

Bacterial organisms in soil can also be used as probiotics. There is evidence, however, that these probiotics can be harmful. Safety of soil-based organisms (SBOs) is a key concern for many healthcare professionals. We share their concern. "Soil-based probiotics can be very easily contaminated with pathogenic strains," explains Lise Alschuler, ND, author and naturopathic oncologist. "In anyone with gastrointestinal distress or illness, these multiple soil-based strains pose risk."

It's interesting to note that some antibiotics have been developed from soil organisms. However, the most notorious soil-based organism is anthrax. Anthrax is a strain of *bacillus* bacteria. *Bacillus* is a common species used in SBOs. Some *bacillus* strains are harmful, as in the case of anthrax, and some are beneficial. The danger is that strains in this particular species can be hard to identify. This can cause a rogue harmful bacteria to make its way into the probiotic product.

Another problem with *bacillus* is that some of the strains interfere with antibiotics. For this reason, it is best to avoid taking SBOs while on antibiotics. This is not the case with other probiotics.

As a result of *bacillus* ingestion, there have been reports of food poisoning and infections. In addition, a Finnish research team determined that *Bacillus licheniformis* added to animal feed caused antibiotic resistance.

In 2004, researchers from the University of London found that while the *baccillus* species showed evidence of colonization, immune stimulation, and antimicrobial activity, they also produced toxins that made them "unsafe for human use." More research involving SBOs is needed before we can fully determine their efficacy and safety.

uses carefully selected all-natural vegetables, fruits, mushrooms, and seaweeds that are placed in the mixture at special times of the year when the ingredient is seasonally ripe. Other probiotics use synthetically created prebiotics that are produced by adding fungal enzymes to white cane sugar.

Natural prebiotics known as oligosaccharides and fructooligosaccharides (FOS) provide nutrients to the lactic acid bacteria and help support the body's production of its innate lactic acid bacteria. FOS is also important in the fermentation process because it strengthens the good bacteria so they are more likely to stick to the colon. FOS refers to a naturally-occurring class of non-digestible carbohydrates or sugars found in foods and plants. Being non-digestible is important because that means they pass through the stomach virtually unchanged. That way they can reach the colon intact so they can be "eaten" by the friendly bacteria. Being non-digestible also means they provide virtually no calories.

Not all forms of FOS are health promoting. Artificial sweeteners, for example, are considered an FOS. Studies have determined that these artificial sweeteners (primarily aspartame) are harmful to our health. There is some speculation that artificial sweetener consumption can contribute to the development of brain disorders, especially in children. There is also some discussion in the scientific community that aspartame may contribute to cancer. However, this connection has not been proven conclusively in humans.

The preferred form of FOS are short-chain oligosaccharides such as molasses and chicory root. Dr. Ohhira's Probiotic 12 PLUS contains only naturally occurring short-chain oligosaccharides. According to a 2006 report in the *Nutrition Journal*, a study involving 200 healthy volunteers demonstrated that by adding short-chain fructo-oligosaccharides to the diet, *bifidobacteria* (a good bacteria) increased significantly.

Some research has demonstrated that prebiotics, in the form of FOS alone without probiotics, help create a positive bacterial balance and promote gut health. Recent research from the University of Milan in Italy demonstrated that FOS helped reduce incidence of allergic reactions and infections in infants during the first two years of life. Because FOS pass through the gut undigested and are fermented in the colon, they enhance the activity of beneficial *bifidobacteria* strains that are already living there.

In addition to feeding our friendly bacteria, prebiotics help encourage important enzyme activity. In order for our good bacteria to thrive, they also depend on enzymes, amino acids, vitamins, and minerals.

Enzymes, amino acids, and more

In the body, an enzyme is a protein that is involved in taking things apart or building things up. For example, enzymes that aid with digestion help break down the foods we eat. Enzymes also help cells grow and help control chemical reactions in the body. Here are just a few examples of enzymes and their actions:

- People who are lactose intolerant have a deficiency of the intestinal enzyme lactase.
- Pancreatic enzymes such as amylase, lipase, and trypsin perform a variety of digestive functions.
- When the heart muscle becomes damaged, the dying cells release enzymes such as creatine kinase and lactic acid dehydrogenase into the blood stream.

Proteolytic enzymes are protein-digesting enzymes that provide a wide range of benefit. In addition to helping with digestion, enzymes help control inflammation and influence our immune system.

Enzymes created during the fermentation of probiotics help enhance digestion and overall health. Some enzymes are made in the stomach, and bacteria can also make important enzymes. Certain bacteria can produce nearly three times as many enzymes as the stomach. For example, while the stomach secretes 99 different enzymes to help break down starch molecules, the bacteria *bacterioides theta* that live in the gut can produce nearly 250 different digestive enzymes. In essence, without friendly bacteria, we can't properly digest food.

Enzymes are important, but so are amino acids—the building blocks of proteins. Amino acids help build new tissue and replace damaged tissue. They help synthesize enzymes, hormones, and hemoglobin (the protein molecule in red blood). There are 10 amino acids that are considered essential. They are essential because we cannot make these amino acids in the body so we must get them from our diet or dietary supplements. The 10 essential amino acids are arginine, histidine, isoleucine, leucine, lysine, methionine, phenylananine, threonin, tryptophan, and valine.

"In addition to prebiotics," explains Dr. Ohhira, "amino acids, vitamins, and minerals provide important supportive factors to lactic acid bacteria." He says, "to achieve the best results, the combination of all of these factors is important."

Is it really possible to get enzymes, amino acids, vitamins, and minerals and viable friendly bacteria from just one probiotic supplement? It is if the probiotic is a synbiotic.

Future looks bright

Probiotic supplementation is important. Don't settle for the cheapest product or the first product you find. Get guidance from someone who knows what to look for in a probiotic supplement. The next chapter provides more detail as to how to choose the best probiotic supplement.

CHAPTER 6

GOING BEYOND PROBIOTICS

PROBIOTICS ARE NO LONGER thought of as "hippie food." Popularity of these dietary supplements has grown far beyond the natural health shopper. In fact, conventional medical doctors, pharmacists, and researchers throughout the United States are finally paying close attention to probiotics.

According to a 2006 report in the *Journal of Pediatric Gastroenterology and Nutrition*, "The use of probiotics, once discussed primarily in the context of alternative medicine, is now entering mainstream medicine." And the impact on the marketplace is astounding.

A recent ABC News report stated that by mid-2008, more than 150 probiotic commercial food products were introduced in the United States. Just three years earlier, there were only 40 new products. In 2006, total sales of probiotic foods and supplements reached nearly $700 million. Analysts at Frost and Sullivan say probiotic food and supplement sales could reach $1.7 billion by 2013.

Probiotics are part of a hot, new category of functional foods. Some health-conscious consumers would rather eat their nutrients than take pills. It seems as though Americans are drawn to foods "spiked" with probiotics. Food manufacturers have been quick to create cute bacterial names like "L casei immunitas" or "bifidus regularis" trying to drive home the fact that beneficial bacterial will boost your immune system and ease digestive woes.

To satisfy the voracious consumer appetite for friendly bacteria, manufacturers are adding the little critters to everything from infant formula to smoothies, snack bars to cereal. Some manufacturers are even trying to boost the bugs in our cheese. And even chocolate lovers can jump on the bacterial bandwagon.

Some food analysts have compared probiotics to oat bran. Remember when it was discovered that oat bran lowered cholesterol? In short order, it seemed as though oat bran was added to everything! Are probiotics this decade's oat bran, as some analysts have said? Just like the good bugs in your gut, this trend needs to have some staying power if we are to experience the benefits of probiotics.

But it's not enough to simply sprinkle some friendly bacteria on your cereal or mix it in your frozen yogurt. In order for probiotics to be effective, there needs to be a structured plan as to how we will repopulate our friendly bacteria beyond the shotgun approach promoted by mass market food manufacturers. If functional foods are your key source of probiotics, just two cautionary notes:

1. Be sure the foods you choose are not high in sugar, additives, and preservatives; choose only all-natural, organic products.
2. Be consistent. Just as a dietary supplement needs to be taken daily, so do your probiotic functional foods.

We do not recommend using probiotic functional foods as your only source of good bacteria. We find that consumers are not getting enough of the friendly bacteria with these foods and that some of these foods can add unwanted calories to the diet. We recommend taking a quality probiotic supplement and only using probiotic foods to fill in potential gaps. Unfortunately, that's not as easy as it sounds.

As we have discussed, probiotics have a lot to offer. But sadly, not all probiotics are created equal. According to Ioannis Misopoulos, Executive Director of the International Probiotics Association (IPA), there is an increasing amount of substandard products being introduced into the United States marketplace. Misopoulos says "A lot of products over promise and under deliver."

A 2006 product evaluation by ConsumerLab.com showed that 44 percent of the products they tested contained fewer viable organisms or low levels of the organisms than claimed by the manufacturers.

As the probiotic business booms, so does the number of probiotic products. To determine if you are getting the probiotic product or food that is most effective, you need to ask the following questions:

- What is the source of the beginning material that created the probiotic?
- How is the probiotic created?
- Is the product guaranteed to deliver viable bacteria until its expiration date, rather than at the time of manufacture?
- Is the product recommended by physicians or healthcare professionals you trust?

Research on probiotics is growing at a rapid pace. Looking at the scientific literature definitely demonstrates why probiotics are so popular, and why more doctors and pharmacists are recommending them now more than ever before.

Scientific credibility

Probiotics and prebiotics are some of the most widely studied natural substances found in the scientific literature. The scientific interest in this area has expanded dramatically. Many highly respected universities throughout the world are interested in probiotics and their impact on health. Even the National Institutes of Health has created the Human Microbiome Project, an important scientific collaboration to evaluate bacteria.

As a result of increased scientific interest, the focus of probiotic research has changed and broadened. There are numerous human double-blinded controlled clinical trials involving probiotics. This type of research is considered the "gold standard" often used by pharmaceutical companies. There is extensive research demonstrating that probiotics are effective in relieving the following gut issues:

- nearly all types of diarrhea;
- constipation;
- gas and bloating;
- irritable bowel disorders; and
- irritable bowel syndrome.

However, probiotic research is no longer confined to digestive and bowel disorders. "Probiotics and prebiotics have long been appreciated for their positive influences on gut health," concluded French researchers in a 2007 article in the journal *Nutrition Review*. "Research on the mechanisms and effects of these agents shows that their impact reaches beyond the intestine."

Some of the areas of interest to researchers include obesity, allergies, skin disorders, and bone health. In 2007, a review by German researchers with the Institute of Physiology and Biochemistry of Nutrition found that prebiotics, in particular, demonstrated bone-building potential in human studies. The researchers concluded that prebiotics have a positive effect on "mineral absorption and metabolism, and bone composition and architecture."

Published research has shown that probiotics can benefit individuals with eczema. In 2007, research from the University of Turku in Finland demonstrated that, by adding *Lactobacillus rhamnosus GG* to infant formula, eczema and allergies in infants were reduced dramatically. We will discuss the wide range of health benefits of probiotics in more detail in Chapter 10.

As we mentioned in Part One, the Human Microbiome Project will also help advance our scientific knowledge of good bacteria, as well as harmful bacteria. The mere fact that we are embarking on such a project is scientifically significant. In the past, all of our efforts have

Dangers of Dairy

Many probiotics, especially in the area of functional foods, are dairy-based. This provides challenges for people who are vegan or lactose intolerant. The vegan diet is totally plant based and does not include dairy. Lactose intolerant people cannot metabolize the sugar found in milk and dairy products. An enzyme in the small intestines known as lactase breaks down these sugar molecules. When there is not enough of this enzyme, the result is mild to severe stomach discomfort. Symptoms include gas, cramping, loose stools or diarrhea, bloating, and/or vomiting which can occur anywhere from 30 minutes to two hours after consuming dairy products. For more information, visit www.lactoseinterolerant.org.

Many people unknowingly have dairy sensitivities. New research has found that dairy can even trigger autistic behavior in children. In susceptible individuals, dairy seeps into the blood stream undigested and attaches to opiate receptors in the brain, which can cause numerous problems associated with behavior and cognition. Researchers from The University of Texas Health Science Center at Houston have found that many children with autism have gastrointestinal problems, and when dairy is avoided they function at a higher level and symptoms subside.

People who have celiac disease or are gluten intolerant should also avoid dairy-based probiotics. These individuals can benefit dramatically by taking a probiotic, but is important that they choose a dairy-free product.

Dairy-based probiotics also need to be refrigerated. Some researchers have called into question the stability and long-term viability of dairy-based friendly bacteria. Also, because of the refrigeration issue, dairy-based probiotics can be inconvenient for travelers.

been placed on researching new antibiotics to kill bacteria. This shift is definitely a step in the right direction.

There are significant and important worldwide efforts being made to positively maximize our relationship with friendly bacteria. Just as the Human Microbiome Project is faced with many challenges, conventional bacterial research has struggled with many issues over the years. For one thing, it's hard to know where to begin. The human body is made up of trillions of bacteria with hundreds of different strains. How do we know which ones to target to show which ones will provide optimum benefit? Also, as discussed in Part One, bacteria are not used to living in a petri dish in isolation. How can we effectively apply that data from the lab to the human body? There are many factors to consider when analyzing friendly bacteria. The first important factor is the starting material or the environment in which the bacteria is created.

Off to a great start

Just as with any friendship, it's important to start out on the right foot. This is also true with our bacterial friends. To get off to a great start with your bacterial buddies, we need to get back to basics. Where do the friendly bacteria actually come from?

Creating proper bacterial balance is like remodeling your house with the help of a few billion friends. We are going to teach you that you can actually remodel your gut. As you know, when you begin any remodeling project, not only is it nice to have help, you need to start with a strong foundation. The quality of your probiotic supplement will determine the strength of your bacterial foundation. Your probiotic supplement can dictate whether your remodeling project will be a huge success or a costly failure.

Japanese researcher Iichiroh Ohhira, PhD, has found that the strongest foundation for our friendly bacteria begins with a whole-foods, natural, and organic diet. Dr. Ohhira artfully combines wild-crafted vegetables, fruits, seaweeds, and mushrooms—92 natural whole food ingredients in all. Wild crafting is when plants are gathered from their natural habitat. These natural ingredients, combined with the potent bacterial strain that he discovered—*Enterococcus faecalis* TH10 from tempeh—is the foundation that Dr. Ohhira builds upon. (To read our interview with Dr. Ohhira, refer to page 98 in Chapter 7.)

Most other probiotics get their start in a petri dish. They are made and put into "bacteria banks" for manufacturers to purchase and put in their products. These bacteria are removed from their cultured medium prior to freeze-drying and/or centrifugation. We'll discuss these manufacturing processes in more detail in the next section. Even if superior strains of bacteria are chosen, the processing of these bacteria can damage them and potentially destroy their chains and colonies. Processing also removes their source of nutrients and protection, which is the culture medium. During processing these "naked" bacteria are then exposed to their worst enemies, light and heat. Their chance for survival following manufacturing is significantly reduced. In addition, many probiotic manufacturers add fillers and sugars, which can further negatively affect the viability of the good bacteria.

Dr. Ohhira's process is a full-culture medium that protects the bacteria from light and heat. These bacteria remain in the comfort and safety of their culture, which also provides nourishment. No violent, damaging process is used. This way the bacteria have a much greater chance of being effective after ingestion.

The most effective probiotic recipe requires meticulous attention to detail. A really great chef pays close attention to the ingredients. But how the product is cooked and for how long is equally important. Growing friendly bacteria is like baking the perfect soufflé. This stage of the probiotic process is called fermentation. How the probiotic is grown will determine if it is a masterpiece or a flop.

As we learned in Part One, famed scientist Louis Pasteur found that fermentation was a biologically active process carried out by microorganisms. As the bacteria starts to break down substances into smaller pieces, the fermentation process begins. Let's take a closer look.

Growing bacteria

All kinds of cells are grown in the lab to help researchers determine how they act—and in some cases, such as with cancer cells, how they can be killed. The medium in which the cells are grown refers to the liquid or gel that is put in the petri dish with the cells. For example, viruses require other living cells in order for them to grow. Human and animal tissue cells often require the addition of hormones or growth factor cells. Bacteria, on the other hand, require nutrients to grow. One way of growing bacteria in the lab is by placing the bacteria in a nutrient mixture or "broth." Sometimes a solid medium or gel substance is used to grow the bacteria.

But how do friendly bacteria make their way into your dietary supplement? After the bacteria are grown, they are placed in a vat and either freeze-dried, spun, pressurized into a powder, or left to ferment over a period of years. Here is a description of these four common manufacturing processes:

- **Freeze-drying:** In a vacuum, using lightening fast speed, the bacteria mixture is exposed to extremes of heat and cold. With freeze-drying, the hope is that when the powder absorbs water again, the bacteria become activated after they are ingested. We do know that some bacteria are damaged during this process, but we don't know how extensive the damage is prior to packaging.

- **Centrifugation:** This spins the bacterial mixture at very high speeds. The bacteria are then forced to congregate to create the substance that goes into the supplement. However, there are many problems with this common technique. First of all, it can separate the bacterial colonies, hampering their viability after ingestion. Second, this process not only damages the bacterial cell, it can break their links to each other and kill them completely.

- **Ultrafiltration:** This method uses a pressure-driven, membrane-based separation process to isolate the bacteria. While it is not as intrusive and dangerous for the bacteria as centrifugation, we do know that some bacterial chains are broken, and the activity and viability of the bacterial colonies is reduced during this process.

- **Natural fermentation:** This occurs when the starting material of bacteria and prebiotics are left to ferment naturally in normal temperatures for a period of years. The finished product is a paste that is then encapsulated in an enteric vegan soft capsule. To our knowledge, the only manufacturer that uses this fermentation process is Dr. Ohhira.

A powder or paste substance is not always encapsulated for use. A good example of this is a common food, such as yogurt, smoothies, or cheese, that is merely spiked with a billion or so bacteria. Sometimes manufacturers also add stabilizers, preservatives, and additives, which makes it even more difficult—and less natural—for the bacteria to survive and thrive.

One of the challenges when buying probiotics or ingesting them in foods is that the manufacturer does not have to tell you how the bacteria got into the capsule or food in the first place. Some manufacturers fully disclose this information, but others do not. Knowing how the bacteria are created is important.

Let's review

We've discussed a lot about probiotics so far. Let's do a quick review of the most salient points:

- It's valuable to know how the bacteria are created and where they come from.

- CFUs are important, but it is not nearly as important as whether or not the bacteria are viable after you ingest them.
- Friendly bacteria need to be surrounded by other friendly bacteria and they need food (prebiotics).
- Beneficial bacteria are taking their rightful place in conventional and respected research circles.
- Consumer interest in probiotics is exploding.

It looks like probiotics have a very bright future. But why take our word for it exclusively? The next chapter features bacteria information from leading experts throughout the world. Let's find out what the future holds for our billion best friends.

7

FUTURE OF PROBIOTICS

A CONVERSATION ABOUT BACTERIA WITH most people has a typical beginning: "Oh yuck, I'm afraid of bacteria!" After explaining that not all bacteria are bad and mentioning the term probiotic, many will respond, "Oh, you mean acidophilus?" Well, not quite, but it's a step in the right direction.

We've seen an important shift. Mainstream news sources are beginning to tell people that not all bacteria are bad. We are finally getting past the fear-based mentality that surrounds our view of bacteria.

Scientific research to date has confirmed that we can successfully join forces with the good bugs in our bodies to help alleviate illness and enhance our overall vitality and wellbeing. But is that the end of the story? Actually, that's just the beginning.

To gain a more comprehensive perspective of this topic, we've searched out some of the leading bacteria experts throughout the world. Our quest for knowledge begins in Japan.

Interview with Iichiroh Ohhira, PhD

For nearly three decades distinguished professor and Japanese research scientist Iichiroh Ohhira, PhD, has been analyzing bacteria. Dr. Ohhira is an award-winning scientist who holds three different doctorate degrees. He is a member of the prestigious New York Academy of Science and serves as the technical advisor on agricultural and environmental issues to the Government of Chengdu, Sichuan Province, China. He has authored or co-authored more than 20 published scientific studies on lactic acid bacteria. His discovery of the proprietary strain *E aecalis* TH10 has been proven to be more than six times stronger than any other naturally-occurring lactic acid bacteria. He is the first person in the world to successfully encapsulate 12 strains of live friendly bacteria in one capsule. We had the rare opportunity to have an in-depth interview with Dr. Ohhira.

Q. What are the main focus areas of your research?

A. I have three main areas of research including anti-allergy; the promotion of chemical-free organic farming and fruit cultivation, including the prevention of continuous cropping-related problems; and research into chemical-free golf courses. All of our research includes the exploration of lactic acid bacteria and how we can more effectively utilize these useful microorganisms.

Q. It seems as though you have a strong interest in the environment and natural health. Does this influence your research direction?

A. Yes. I have always been interested in agriculture and natural sciences. I studied microbiology, specifically lactic acid bacteria, at Okayama University in Japan with Professor Nakae, a world authority. I am interested in learning new things and teaching others. I have always known that we should have respect for our environment and that the source of the foods we eat is as important as the foods themselves. My interest in the environment and agriculture led me to lactic acid bacteria. I soon discovered that these useful microorganisms are essential to health.

Q. What are some of the significant discoveries you and your research team have made?

A. Certainly the discovery of *Enterococcus faecalis* TH10 was significant and our research on its antimicrobial activity against MRSA. More broadly, in the 1980s, we discovered that more lactic acid bacteria are not necessarily better. Most research in other countries has focused on inundating the body with large numbers of colony forming units of one or two strains. Our research showed us that flooding the body in this way can activate the body's T and B cells to fight what they perceive as invading bad bacteria. In other words, this strategy was causing the opposite effect of what we wanted from lactic acid bacteria.

Q. When you found this out, what did you do?

A. We focused on ways to support the individual strains in the human body. Of course, we don't know exactly what strains are in each individual, so we needed to find a way to enhance the body's capabilities to produce its own unique strains of lactic acid bacteria and then help those bacteria become strong and repopulate.

Q. How did you do this?

A. We began by researching the best way to encourage the growth of live and viable strains of lactic acid bacteria. We found that we needed several strains, not just one or two, and we knew we needed to encourage their growth in a natural setting. So, after much experimenting, we came up with a proprietary blend of wild-crafted fruits, herbs, and seaweeds. We found that the most effective recipe includes a blend of 92 natural crops including herbs, fruits, roots, vegetables, and mushrooms. We also add the *E faecalis TH10* bacteria from tempeh, which is a traditional fermented delicacy from Malaysia.

We discovered that a multi-year, normal temperature, natural fermentation process is necessary. We don't just take all 92 crops and throw them in a vat to ferment. We introduce each ingredient when it is seasonally ripe. This assures productive fermentation. We found that certain ingredients should be introduced only in a specific season—fall, winter, spring, or summer.

Q. Why is it important to ferment for such a long time?

A. The longer the fermentation, the more powerful and viable the lactic acid bacteria will become. This process allows the weaker bacteria to die off and the stronger bacteria to become even stronger. Through natural selection, the bacteria gain strength with each generation through each season. Only time can provide this benefit.

Q. Why is this important?

A. If the bacteria are not strong when they are packaged, there is less of a chance they will survive. They need to survive packaging and shipping, but they also need to survive once they are ingested. We have found that after ingestion, the TH10 strain resides in the gastrointestinal tract for an extended period of time where it flourishes and co-exists with the individual's colonizing bacteria, like the *lactobacillus* and *bifidobacteria* strains that already inhabit the intestinal walls.

Q. How does this compare to other methods of probiotic preparation, such as freeze drying, centrifuging, or ultrafiltration?

A. Friendly bacteria grow in a cultured medium, which is a solution that contains all of the nutrients that the bacteria need to grow. As the bacteria grow, they transform the culturing medium into a different substance. This is a completely new compound that contains everything necessary for the bacteria to thrive. The processing methods you mention separate this new substance and destroy the best condition for the friendly bacteria to survive and provide health benefits. The addition of stabilizers, preservatives, and pasteurization will further weaken the lactic acid bacteria. The fermentation process that I have developed maintains the integrity of the whole versus isolating the bacterial parts. Lactic acid bacteria must be viable in order to be effective. In addition, they need organic acids, micronutrients, and natural prebiotics in order to thrive.

Q. Why are organic acids, micronutrients, and natural prebiotics important?

A. Because it provides food for the lactic acid bacteria. Just as we require food to live, so do bacteria. The recipe we have chosen, which ferments for at least three years, is specifically designed to keep the lactic acid bacteria viable for a longer period of time. These prebiotics feed the probiotics.

Q. It sounds like an arduous task?

A. It is, but it is the only way. We must be vigilant about the addition of the natural ingredients and the bacterial strains. We must be patient if we are to achieve the results we desire.

Let's continue our quest for bacterial information in Ireland.

Interview with Eamonn Quigley, MD

Gastroenterology is an important sub-specialty in medicine. As digestive disorders become increasingly common, it is the role of the gastroenterologist to stay abreast of scientific advancements in the areas of diagnosis and treatment. Because bacteria are the main "residents" of the gastrointestinal system, this is becoming a key area of focus for this important medical specialty.

One of the leading gastroenterologists in the world is Eamonn Quigley, MD. Dr. Quigley is the president of the World Gastroenterology Organization and the American College of Gastroenterology. He is Professor of Medicine and Human Physiology at the University College Cork in Cork, Ireland. After graduating from the University College Cork, Dr. Quigley spent some time in the United Kingdom, specifically in Glasgow and Manchester, and in the United States at the Mayo Clinic and at the University of Nebraska Medical Center. While at Nebraska, he developed a clinical research center in gastro-intestinal motility and correlated clinical studies with both in vitro (test tube) and in vivo (animal) models. In 1998, he returned to Cork. Dr. Quigley has published more than 400 original articles, reviews, editorials, and book chapters. He has also co-authored or authored six books and monographs on the topic of gastroenterology.

In 2007, Dr. Quigley told the *Internal Medicine World Report* that the field of probiotics is "now beyond the threshold in terms of a major breakthrough."

Q. **Why are you interested in the science of bacteria and how do you feel about the Human Microbiome Project?**

A. Because the intestinal flora and how it interacts with the host [humans] in health and disease is of tremendous importance. This is a new frontier in medical science and one that will have tremendous impact. I am extremely enthusiastic about the Human Microbiome Project as it promises to reveal the true magnitude and diversity of the human microbiota, which has been grossly underestimated by conventional culture techniques.

Q. **As probiotics gain more widespread acceptance and their use increases, do you have any concerns?**

A. I have several concerns, mostly related to quality control. No two probiotics are alike. Attempts to promote one particular probiotic on the basis of evidence generated in the study of another probiotic may be completely unfounded, and even bogus. Similarly, those who fail to provide well-substantiated data on the actual species and strains, bacterial numbers, viability in the long-term, the conditions in which the product is stored, and efficacy based on controlled clinical trials of their product should remain suspect. All claims must be substantiated by good data. On the safety side, there also must be good data to ensure the product is completely safe for human consumption.

Q. What are some of the biggest misconceptions about probiotics?

A. That all probiotics are the same and they are all equally effective or useless.

Q. How do we address this misconception?

A. The only way to counteract this belief is through good physician- and scientist-led education. We also need better regulation of the probiotic products being marketed. This may surprise you, but some of us working in this area would welcome more regulation.

Q. Are there advances in testing techniques that will help determine the therapeutic efficacy of probiotics?

A. There are rapidly evolving techniques in genomics, metabolomics, metagenomics, and immunology. We are continuing to receive emerging data from these fields that will help guide us in this area. We are also gaining a better understanding of the immunology of the flora-host interaction. This will be fundamental to defining, understanding, and comparing probiotic action, efficacy, and safety.

Q. **How will probiotics become incorporated more fully into the gastroenterology medical specialty?**

A. They will be incorporated on the basis of good science and following more quality clinical research. The field of gastroenerlogy shows much greater enthusiasm for probiotics than in the past. There is more acceptance of probiotics, not just within this medical specialty, but in medicine in general. New potential roles for probiotics include the prevention and/or treatment of allergy, obesity, and liver disease.

The North American perspective

We've had the opportunity to talk to many healthcare professionals about this important topic. Gregor Reid, PhD, Professor of Microbiology at the University of Western Ontario in Canada, is a leading researcher in the field. Dr. Reid's focus is on how probiotics can be used to help women, including those with repeated vaginal infections, subject to premature babies, or who have or are at risk of HIV infection. We asked Dr. Reid to identify his primary concern about the growing interest in probiotics.

"There are too many companies selling probiotics that are not even probiotics," he explained. "These products have never been tested on humans or shown to provide benefit. This could severely hurt the field." Dr. Reid concludes, "However, because it is proven that our bodies benefit from lactic acid bacteria, we should not be afraid to try some for a few months."

Pharmacy is one area where probiotic use can be especially beneficial. It is our hope that, in the future, when a doctor writes a prescription for an antibiotic, there will be directions on how and when to take a probiotic. For now, this burden largely falls on the shoulders of holistic medical doctors and integrative pharmacists like Ross Pelton, RPh.

Pelton recommends probiotics specifically for those who have been on a course of antibiotics; babies born cesarean; newborn babies who are not breastfed; anyone taking medications that interfere with normal GI function, such as antacids, anti-ulcer, and GERD medications; and anyone experiencing symptoms of gastrointestinal problems. We asked Pelton what he felt the biggest misconceptions consumers have about probiotics.

"Most people do not understand the importance of quality when it comes to probiotic products," he said. "Many people will tend to grab the least expensive product on the shelf of a pharmacy or health food store. Many people do not understand the power, importance, and significance of a specialized therapeutic probiotic."

Pelton explains that most of the people he encounters are confused about bacterial strains. He says, "People see claims being made for a particular strain of probiotic based on a study and then they think they can purchase just any probiotic to get the same results as the study." Of course, that's not the case.

Best-selling author and nutritionist Ann Louise Gittleman, PhD, CNS, utilizes probiotics as one of the focal parts of her popular Gut Flush Plan. "Make sure your probiotic contains bacterial strains known to destroy the Superbugs," explained Gittleman. For example, she says "*Enterococcus faecalie* TH10 was fermented and isolated over a five-year period, resulting in a super probiotic strain potent enough to destroy MRSA, as well as *salmonella, E. coli*, and *H. pylori*."

National Institutes of Health

In 2007, Alan Krensky, MD, was named the first NIH Deputy Director for the Office of Portfolio Analysis and Strategic Initiatives. This new office is designed to explore new, cutting edge areas of research. After a year-long process, the Human Microbiome Project was identified as one of the most important, innovative research areas. It is a direct offshoot of the Human Genome Project. Dr. Krensky plays a key leadership role at the NIH. He is a member of the American

Society for Clinical Investigation and the Association of American Physicians and is a co-author of more than 260 research papers. He is also an award-winning scientist with interests in human cellular and molecular immunology, as well as transplantation and tumor immunology. We had the opportunity to interview Dr. Krensky after he had been in his position for about 18 months. [Editor's Note: Dr. Krenksy has since left his position as Deputy Director for the Office of Portfolio Analysis and Strategic Initiatives. He continues to do research in immunology.]

Q. Why is there now so much interest in bacteria?

A. The fact that we are more microbial than we are human catches attention. Bacterial cells significantly outnumber our "human" cells, and what excites researchers is that they are here for a reason. We would like to find out how much they impact who we are, what we are, how we work, and how we feel.

Q. Why is the Microbiome Project at the top of the list when it comes to key areas of research?

A. The work from Dr. Jeffrey Gordon at Washington University and other groups really caught the public eye. Their research showed that microbes can make a fat mouse thin or vice versa. That information got into the lay press and was very newsworthy. The Microbiome Project hopes to discover if microbes really impact whether we are fat or thin, happy or sad, healthy or sick. In the past, the only way we could find out anything about microbes was to grow them. As a result of the Human Genome Project, we have new technologies that didn't exist in the past. We now have sophisticated sequencing techniques that will allow us to find out a lot more about bacteria. It's a whole new world. The germ theory was totally transformative, and gave rise to antibiotics and how we do surgery. The Human Microbiome Project will be just as transformative.

Q. What is the most significant aspect of the Human Microbiome Project?

A. It follows the model of the Human Genome Project, which is unprecedented collaboration. A lot of good science happens in individual laboratories with smart people and good ideas. But we are in a new era where we can use technology, databases, and a variety of different people with different backgrounds that come together. This is team science at it's best that is completely technology oriented. It is also an international collaboration. We have already joined forces with the European Union. China, Japan, Australia, and Canada are also very interested. NIH is taking a leadership role, but this is definitely a collaboration and data sharing. This will be significant because we will be able to show how the environment, as well as personal genetics, plays a role. The more diversified the data, the better.

We are also making a significant financial investment of $115 million. That's a lot of money that the American tax-payers are paying to learn about this important new area. We believe the pay off will be incredible and have huge positive health implications.

The wrong direction

Thanks to the advances in scientific research, countless lives have been saved. We can transplant many major organs of the human body and even give someone a new heart if they need it. Technological marvels in medicine can help an amputee walk again, locate hard-to-find cancers, and allow us to consistently measure blood sugar with just a prick of the finger. We can make new skin for burn victims and help people hear, see, and even think better. There is no question that medical science is not only fascinating, it can be life-changing.

But medical science, and more specifically food science, is not without its dark side. Case in point, genetically modified organisms

(GMOs). Shockingly, about 70 percent of our food supply is from genetically modified sources. You were probably not even aware of this fact because the FDA does not require GMO information to appear on food labels. We feel this is wrong. We would like to be given the choice to eat GMO foods. However, if it's not listed on the label, we can't make that informed decision. If you feel the same way, you can visit www.responsibletechnology.org for more information. To avoid GMOs, choose organic foods whenever possible (for more information on organics, refer to the side bar on page 41).

There are many production advantages to modifying the genetic make up of a food:

- longer shelf life;
- quicker growing time;
- bigger animals; and
- more milk.

As a result of all of these "advantages," we were promised lower food costs. Did we miss something? Food costs in our neighborhoods are going up! If those are the advantages, what are the disadvantages?

According to the US Government (yes, the same one that approved these foods), there are several concerns associated with GMOs including:

- increased incidence of allergies;
- antibiotic resistance (we don't need more of that!);
- unknown long-term effects (because there have been no clinical safety trials done);
- contamination and cross-pollination of other crops; and
- loss of flora biodiversity in the soil and in ourselves (that's a BIG step backwards).

To us, the disadvantages far outweigh any perceived advantages. But how did so many of these GMO foods sneak their way into our food supply without having clinical trials done on safety? According to the FDA, they didn't think it was necessary and they thought

Genetically-Modified Mess

Sometimes we can be a bit overzealous in our efforts to take something good and make it better. This is the case with genetically-modified organisms (GMOs). According to the National Organic Standards Board, "GMOs are made with techniques that alter the molecular or cell biology of an organism by means that are not possible under natural conditions or processes." GMOs and their derivatives are prohibited in organic food production and handling systems. The Organic Trade Association concludes, "The use of GMOs is an uproven technology and one that an organic agricultural system does not need in order to grow high quality and nutritious food."

Ingestion of GMO foods can cause allergies and issues of antibiotic resistance. Long-term damage to our health and our environment is unknown at this time. In addition to the potential negative health effects, farming with GMOs is not good for the environment. Due to cross contamination, GMO farming can also negatively impact organic farming efforts. For more information on organic farming visit www.ota.com. We suggest buying local, non-GMO foods whenever possible. In addition to being healthier for you, it will also help support your local farming community.

it would be too difficult to do. What would happen if we took that same attitude about drugs? This is our food supply—something far more important!

What's in store for us in the future regarding GMO foods? According to the US Government, there will be "bananas that produce human vaccines against infectious diseases such as hepatitis B, fish that mature more quickly, and plants that produce plastics with unique properties." That's all we need, virus-infused bananas, fish on steroids, and more plastic.

The GMO craze began with the humble tomato, the first genetically modified food. There is a protein in tomatoes that cause them to get soft as it ripens, just as Mother Nature intended. Unfortunately, for the large tomato growers, this made it hard to transport ripe tomatoes clear across the country. A new gene helped create the Flavr Savr Tomato—plump, yet firm enough to leap tall buildings and travel around the world if necessary. Honestly, we don't want our tomatoes shipped from clear across the country anyway. We buy locally grown tomatoes whenever possible, not just because they taste better but they also help reduce our carbon footprint, which helps the environment.

One may argue that there is one success story regarding GMOs. Golden Rice has more beta-carotene and iron, and is being fed to people in underdeveloped countries that have high incidence of anemia and childhood blindness. Perhaps this is a good idea, but how did we make the leap of creating better rice for starving children to saturating our food supply with these Franken Foods? And what right do we have to experiment on people in underdeveloped countries. The fact is, we don't know the long-term affects of these foods.

Have we gone too far? We think so. At a bare minimum, these foods should be labeled and consumers should be made aware of what they are eating. The European Union is far ahead of us on this one. By last count (2007 figures), Europe had 174 regions declared as GMO-free. Europe has a strong commitment to ban GMOs from their agriculture and food.

What does this have to do with probiotics? You guessed it—genetically modified probiotics are presently in development. Known as "designer probiotics," these substances are presently being aggressively studied. The idea is to make something good even better. But how far will we go? Will we have a repeat performance of the antibiotic debacle that we find ourselves in or the excessive use of GMOs in our food supply?

Researchers at the University College Cork in Ireland are tinkering with specific strains in test tubes to try to create "more technologically robust and effective probiotic cultures." One idea is to use probiotics to develop new vaccines or help with drug delivery. In

2006, research by Charles Elson, MD, from the University of Alabama, studied a bioengineered strain of bacteria on 10 patients with Crohn's disease. It was not effective.

Over the past few years, interest in genetically modified probiotics has been increasing. In some cases, this could be another one of those medical advances that helps many people overcome illness. But if taken too far, this could be devastating to a society that is already stricken with severe issues of bacterial imbalance.

Sure, if we fiddle with something long enough, we will find a way to change it. We may even find a way to make it better. But let's proceed with caution. We asked Dr. Quigley what he thought of designer probiotics. "They may be the way forward in some situations," he said, "but for others, naturally-occurring probiotics may suffice."

Of course, a discussion about the future is not complete without a prediction. We predict that if too much scientific focus is placed on genetically modified probiotics, we will repeat history. Now that we have finally embraced the idea that not all bacteria are bad and, in fact, many bacteria are our "friends," can we be so arrogant to think that we need to change them to more appropriately fit our needs? Yes, there may be applications for these high-tech designer probiotics. Let's first try to figure out what the good bugs in our bodies do first before manipulating them. And of course, let's not mess with Mother Nature too much. She's done a pretty good job so far. She's the one who gave us probiotics in the first place. We are sure she knows what she's doing.

The right direction

Research in the area of probiotics is definitely making progress. Not that long ago, the only characteristic we looked for in a probiotic supplement was the number of bacteria supposedly present at the time of manufacture. Today, we understand that it's not just about quantity, it's about quality.

"Probiotic research has implications for clinical diagnosis of several diseases by testing the flora, sampling the intestinal mucosa, and measuring the systemic immune response to see if the host-flora interaction is appropriate or disturbed," reports the December 2007 issue of *Internal Medical World Report*. "Therapeutic efficacy depends on the ability to modulate disturbed flora or the immune response with probiotics."

Research should continue to focus on learning how beneficial bacteria can contribute to our overall health. Many unanswered questions about probiotics remain. What is the exact dosage required for prevention versus treatment of a specific illness? Which strains provide what benefit? How can we more accurately determine our individual bacterial needs? How exactly do bacteria influence illness?

So far, what we do know is that good bacteria are our allies. Probiotics can help us prevent and treat some of the most uncomfortable and serious illnesses of our time.

As for the future of "designer" probiotics, stay tuned! It will be a story worth following.

Part Three
SOMETHING'S WRONG

8

DIGESTION, ELIMINATION, AND DETOXIFICATION

WE AREN'T SURE WHO COINED the term "Death begins in the colon." Perhaps it was a coroner who had a birds-eye view, or maybe it was a colon hydrotherapist anxious to promote his/her services. No matter who first said it, it is a widely held belief that digestion and the condition of the colon can profoundly impact our overall health. In fact, the developer of the colonoscope, Hiromi Shinya, MD, can tell your biological age from looking at your colon.

It's easy to take the colon and the entire digestive system for granted—until there is a problem. After all, digestion seems like a pretty simple process: Take food in, extract the nutrients, and eliminate everything else. However, the digestive system, technically known as the gastrointestinal system, can be rife with dysfunction and the cause of many medical issues. And when a problem occurs, this sophisticated system tells us loud and clear through a variety of uncomfortable—and sometimes embarrassing—symptoms including gas, bloating, heartburn, diarrhea, constipation, and in more serious cases, disease states such as ulcers, infections, colitis, and cancer. Before we can prevent the plethora of problems associated with digestion, we must first understand its basic operation.

Digestion description

Digestion is a significant physical and chemical process designed to convert food to fuel so we can be healthy, and have energy and nourishment to thrive. Within 24 to 72 hours, the food we eat makes its way through the entire digestive system. The process begins in the mouth with physical chewing and the release of enzymes in our saliva. From there, the food is transported to the stomach where more processing takes place; acid is released into the mix and intrinsic factor (a glycoprotein produced in the stomach) helps to transport vitamin B12 into the small intestine for absorption. The gallbladder then releases bile into the beginning of the small intestine to further help break down the food. After a journey through about 25 feet of small intestines, the partially digested food makes its way to the large intestine. The reason this part of the intestines is called large is because of the diameter, not the length. The extra diameter helps the large intestines transform the remaining material into stool so it can be eliminated. The large intestine is also known as the colon and this is where the waste material becomes dryer so it can be removed via a bowel movement. A healthy bowel movement should occur one to three times a day.

Some very significant actions happen along each step of the digestive process. For example, while the food is in the small intestines, immune cells are released to test the material for bacterial contaminants. If contaminants are found, they are neutralized so they can be safely eliminated. Also nutrients are extracted from food and transported across the intestinal lining into the blood stream. Hormones and the nervous system help regulate this part of the digestive process. The absorption of key nutrients and the elimination of toxic substances are critical functions of healthy digestion.

The majority of bacteria in our bodies are in the colon (at least one billion per milliliter of fluid). The small intestine, on the other hand, has only about 10,000 bacteria per milliliter of fluid. The strains

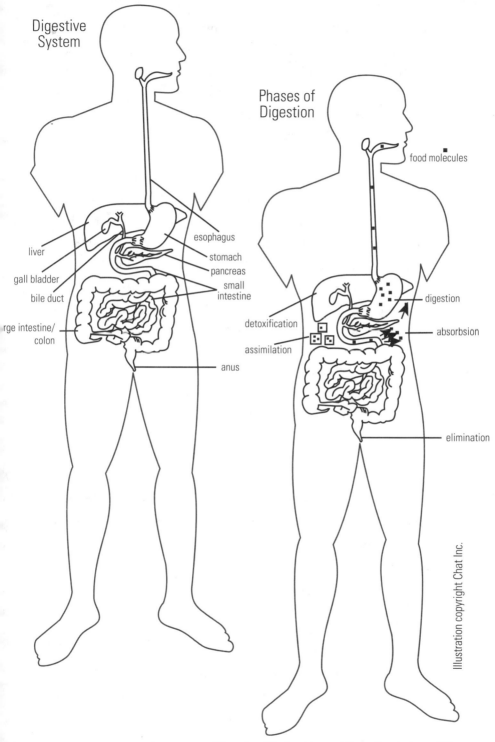

Digestive
System

liver

gall bladder

bile duct

rge intestine/
colon

Phases of
Digestion

esophagus

stomach

pancreas

small
intestine

anus

food molecules

detoxification

assimilation

digestion

absorbsion

elimination

Illustration copyright Chat Inc.

Digestion, Elimination, and Detoxification   117

of bacteria in the colon are completely different than the strains in the small intestine. In cases of bacterial overgrowth or imbalance, the bacteria from the colon spills into the small intestine. Bacterial imbalance is referred to as dysbiosis. Proper bacterial balance is known as eubiosis. Dysbiosis can be dangerous to our health.

As we mentioned, important functions take place in the small intestine. This is where food is broken down and nutrients are extracted and delivered to other parts of the body via the blood. After extraction, these nutrients are transported across the intestinal lining. This is also where the food is tested for bad bacteria and other contaminants. If the small intestine does not have the proper ratio of good to bad bacteria, or the bad bacteria have taken over completely, these two key functions are dramatically disrupted. When this happens, the intestinal lining becomes too thin and the immune response goes into overdrive. If the immune system continues to respond inappropriately, it creates autoimmunity. We'll discuss the immune system in more detail in the next chapter.

When the intestinal lining becomes too thin, there are grave absorption issues. This is known as leaky gut syndrome.

Have I sprung a leak?

What happens when the holes of a colander for cooking are too large or a net becomes worn? Things fall through. This is exactly what happens with leaky gut syndrome. Things—namely food particles, toxins, and other harmful substances—can slip through into the blood stream. The gut becomes "leaky." Keep in mind this is on a microscopic level. We are not able to see these holes with the naked eye or even through a colonoscopy. That is why so many people with digestive issues see a GI specialist and undergo a battery of tests only to be told there is nothing wrong with them.

In order for cells and organs in the human body to function properly, they require nutrients. The purpose of a healthy intestinal lining

Following is a list of symptoms and conditions associated with leaky gut syndrome:

Symptoms

- chronic bad breath
- diarrhea
- constipation
- menstrual issues
- bruising
- hyperactivity
- bloating
- gas
- fatigue
- inability to concentrate
- mood swings
- indigestion
- itchiness
- stuffed or runny nose
- sinus problems
- heart palpitations

Conditions

- acne
- allergies
- arthritis
- asthma
- attention deficit hyperactivity disorder (ADHD)
- bladder infection
- breast cancer
- colon cancer
- prostate cancer
- candidiasis (yeast infection)
- Crohn's disease
- depression and/or anxiety
- eczema
- high cholesterol
- irritable bowel syndrome (IBS)
- liver disease
- osteoporosis
- premenstrual syndrome (PMS)

is to allow properly digested particles from fats, proteins, and carbo-hydrates to pass through it into the blood stream. Those nutrients are then delivered to the cells and nutrients that require them to function properly. In addition, a healthy lining acts as a barrier to keep out dis-ease causing bacteria, foreign substances, and larger undigested food particles that can become problematic. Probiotics ensure the intestinal lining remains healthy by helping to create properly bacterial balance in the intestines. This helps ensure protection against substances that can harm us. It also helps prevent leaky gut syndrome.

When there is a proper balance of good to bad bacteria, the intestinal lining remains strong. It is our internal fortress against invaders. Good bacteria are the soldiers that protect the walls. Through a process known as competitive exclusion, the good bac-teria compete with disease-causing bacteria for food and space on the intestinal lining. When the good bacteria lose the competition, they become overpowered by harmful bacteria, which then starve the good and steal their spot on the lining. This is when the intesti-nal lining becomes damaged. As a result, the irritated and inflamed lining has increased permeability (leaking), allowing all kinds of substances to enter the blood stream that normally would not have gotten through.

Dysbiosis and leaky gut syndrome go hand-in-hand. The over-growth of bad bacteria upset the ecological bacterial balance in the intestines, which in turn damages the intestinal lining. Leo Galland, MD, is a researcher specializing in dysbiosis. He helped create a medical policy to help identify dysbiosis for Oregon, Utah, Idaho, and select counties in Washington State. Galland has found that stool and urine analysis can provide important markers to determine if someone is in a state of dysbiosis. According to a Blue Cross Blue Shield medical policy statement, "Reference laboratories specializ-ing in the evaluation of dysbiosis may offer comprehensive testing of various aspects of digestion, absorption, microbiology, and metabolic

Some Common Harmful Substances

- Hormones in the food supply

- Estrogens in water, plastic, and other substances

- Agricultural pesticides and herbicides

- Genetically modified foods

- Industrial chemicals released into the air, soil, and water

- Ionizing and non-ionizing radiation (microwaves, cell phones, x-rays)

- Smoke and second hand smoke

markers." If you are not in Oregon, Utah, Idaho, or Washington, your doctor may not be familiar with these tests. Naturopathic physicians and holistic-minded medical doctors, however, are receptive to doing these tests. To find a naturopathic physician in your area visit www.naturopathic.org.

Many doctors will test for leaky gut using a system that involves consuming two sugars, mannitol and lactulose. The test looks at the ratio of these two sugars in your urine. If there is a high amount of lactulose in your urine, it indicates that you may have leaky gut syndrome. For information about doctors who do this test visit www.acam.org or call 1-800-532-3688.

Because absorption issues can cause systemic problems throughout the body, symptoms and conditions associated with leaky gut syndrome are extremely varied and may cause a wide spectrum of symptoms and illnesses. Leaky gut can cause mild constipation to severe liver dysfunction. Unexplainable symptoms such as fatigue or depression can be caused by leaky gut. Nearly all chronic digestive disorders can be linked, in part or in whole, to a leaky gut. Arthritis, eczema, and autism, as well as cancer, high cholesterol, osteoporosis, and many other conditions can all be linked to leaky gut syndrome. For a complete list of symptoms and conditions associated with leaky gut, refer to the side bar on page 119.

With such a long list of symptoms and conditions associated with leaky gut, it's not surprising that dysbiosis is also associated with accelerated aging. This is due, in part, to the nutritional deficiencies that come from having a leaky gut. The proper balance of good to bad bacteria will help you feel and look younger. Proper bacterial balance also facilitates efficient elimination and detoxification, critical components of good health.

Elimination and detoxification

Proper elimination and detoxification are the final phases of digestion. Every day we are exposed to harmful substances. We drink them, eat them, and breathe them every moment of our lives. In addition to entering our system through the gastrointestinal tract, toxins can also be absorbed through the skin. We release toxins through feces, urine, sweat, and breath.

It is important to have a bowel movement one to three times per day. If a bowel movement is achieved fewer than three times per week, you may be constipated. Constipation is a symptom, not a disease. Nearly everyone will experience constipation at some point. If constipation becomes chronic and painful, see a doctor.

Several studies have shown that beneficial bacteria can help ease constipation. A 2007 study featured in *Pediatrics International* involving 45 children with chronic constipation demonstrated that probiotics, combined with magnesium oxide, was effective in significantly increasing the number of bowel movements without side effects.

Toxins that are not directly eliminated through feces and urine are sent to the liver for processing. The liver is the most important tool

Bad Belly Bacteria

Breaking down food into energy requires some pretty harsh chemicals. When food enters the stomach, it is sprayed with hydrochloric acid and enzymes. A thick mucous coating that lines the inside of the stomach protects it from this acidic environment. Because these chemicals are so severe, it was believed that nothing could survive in it. And then came along the *H pylori* bacteria, discovered by a couple of Australian researchers in 1982.

H pylori is a spiral shaped bacteria that burrows its way into the mucous membrane of the stomach. Once embedded, it protects itself by secreting its own enzymes that neutralize the enzymes produced in the stomach. A breath test will actually reveal the gases from the enzymes produced by *H pylori*. The body tries to fight *H pylori* by sending white blood cells and other immune cells to the site of the bacteria. Unfortunately, the immune cells cannot easily penetrate the stomach lining to get to the safe mucous membrane. This causes the immune system to continue its relentless pursuit of *H pylori*. The result is inflammation of the stomach lining surrounding the bacteria. This inflammation eventually develops into a sore and then a peptic ulcer.

In 2006, researchers from Stanford University discovered even more bacteria in the stomach. One of the types they discovered is related to *Deinococcus radiodurans*, one of the strongest bacteria ever discovered. It can survive in radioactive waste dumps and hot springs. It is so hardy that scientists have dubbed it "Conan the Bacterium." According to an article by Ker Than of LiveScience, the Stanford researchers "extracted snippets of genetic material from the stomachs of 19 people and found the biological blueprints of 128 bacteria types. Many of them had never been observed in the stomach before and 10 percent were previously unknown to science."

As it turns out, *H pylori* is not the only bacteria in our bellies. The next step is to determine which bacteria live there and which are just passing through. Just as the discovery of *H pylori* in the stomach led to finding out one of the possible causes of ulcers, perhaps we will learn more about these other bacteria and their role in health and disease.

we have in detoxifying harmful chemicals. More than two quarts of blood pass through the liver every minute of every day. The liver filters toxins from the blood and turns them into benign substances that can safely be removed from the body through healthy elimination. In addition, the liver sends bile into the stomach, which helps digest fats. Bile also attaches to toxins so they can be eliminated in feces.

Why is efficient elimination and detoxification so important? We live in a toxic world. Our body has to process toxic chemicals constantly in order to keep us healthy. There are more than 85,000 synthetic chemicals registered in the world. The average home contains anywhere from three to ten gallons of chemical waste. This could be paint, air fresheners, carpet deodorizers, drain cleaners, and the list goes on. Carpeting emits more than 200 chemicals that can end up in the body. There are toxins in plastic, hormones and antibiotic residue in food, and pollution in the air. Municipal drinking water has been shown to be one of the worst culprits. Tap water can contain arsenic, lead, radon, pharmaceuticals and other toxic chemicals.

Many of the synthetic chemicals we are exposed to have been directly linked to a variety of illnesses including brain disorders and cancer. Remember, besides the skin, the digestive system has the most contact with the outside world because of what we eat and drink. Our ability to detoxify chemicals and harmful substances we are exposed to every day is critical.

There are numerous factors that can weaken our detoxification system including:

- nicotine
- alcohol consumption
- prescription and over-the-counter drugs such as acetaminophen, benozodiazepines, antihistamines, and cimetidine
- nutritional deficiencies, specifically iron, and vitamins A and C
- hydrocarbons formed during charcoal grilling

The important role of exercise

A healthy diet should be paired with an active lifestyle. Physical activity can improve our health and the health of our beneficial bacteria on so many levels. Studies have shown that consistent exercise can stimulate the immune system, reduce inflammation, help control insulin resistance, promote healthy digestion and elimination, improve mood and self-esteem, increase oxygen to the brain, and help maintain a healthy weight. As author and clinician Dr. Lise Alschuler says, "It's amazing that something as simple as moving will provide that much benefit."

Here are some key exercise tips to keep in mind:

- Incorporate all three types of exercises into your weekly routine including aerobics (brisk walking, biking, swimming), stretching (yoga, tai chi), and strength training (Pilates, weight lifting).

- Make exercise a part of your regular routine and mix it up to make if fun and prevent boredom.

- Be sure to warm up and cool down with some simple stretching; this will also help enhance flexibility.

- Exercise can be fun if you choose activity you enjoy or maybe even find a "work-out buddy" to help keep you motivated.

- As you get more fit, increase the intensity and duration of your exercise routine.

- Drink plenty of fresh water before, during, and after you work out.

- Consistency and frequency are the keys to a successful exercise program.

If you have been inactive for a long period of time, you should contact your doctor to ensure you are healthy enough to begin exercising.

Natural substances that have been shown to support proper detoxification include:

- probiotics from synergistic lactic acid bacterial strains
- prebiotics from whole food sources
- EGCG from green tea
- indoles from cruciferous vegetables
- carnosol from rosemary
- quercetin from onions and apples
- eugenol from cloves
- capsicum from cayenne
- resveratrol from red grapes
- aged garlic extract

Silymarin extract has been shown in clinical studies to be especially beneficial to proper liver function. Research has shown that silymarin can actually help the liver regenerate. A 2006 research review featured in the *Indian Journal of Medical Research* confirmed that silymarin has a good safety profile and has clinical applications for alcoholic liver, cirrhosis, mushroom poisoning, viral hepatitis, toxic and drug-induced liver disease, and diabetes.

By correcting bacterial imbalance, probiotics also improve the health of the liver. In 2003, researchers from Johns Hopkins University demonstrated that non-alcoholic fatty liver disease (NAFLD) is caused by bacterial imbalance in the gut. In 2006, researchers from the Imperial College of London found that the presence of a specific microbe in mice predisposed them to the development of NAFLD.

Focusing on healthy digestion

A properly functioning digestive system plays a critical role in our overall health and the prevention of serious illness. All of the nutrients needed to sustain life are absorbed through our gastrointestinal tract. If there are problems anywhere along the route, we are not getting the nourishment we need to be healthy. In addition to promoting healthy digestion, we also need a strong immune system and a balanced inflammatory response. Along with digestion and elimination, the operation of these two key body functions will determine whether or not we get sick or stay well. To prevent illness, it's important to understand the causes. The next chapter will explore this important area of health education.

CHAPTER

9

CAUSES OF ILLNESS

AS WE LEARNED IN THE last chapter, issues with digestion will certainly benefit from probiotics and proper bacterial balance. When bad bacteria dominate the digestive system, serious problems can occur including absorption issues, inefficient elimination, and inadequate detoxification. Lack of probiotics has also been shown to increase other significant risk factors associated with the development of disease.

There are some risk factors we cannot control, such as genetics and the environment (e.g., pollution). But there are definitely dietary and lifestyle factors that we can control including:

- eating less sugar;
- reducing alcohol consumption;
- not smoking;
- exercising more; and
- limiting the amount of fermented and yeast-laden foods we eat.

While we cannot change our genetic make up, there are lots of things we can do to prevent illness. The next section outlines our proactive disease prevention plan. Scientific research has clearly shown that if we have a normal weight, strong immune system, an appropriate internal inflammatory response, and stable blood sugar levels, the chance of developing a serious illness is dramatically reduced. As a result, disease prevention should focus on four key areas: reducing obesity, increasing immunity, stabilizing inflammation, and controlling insulin resistance. Bacterial balance plays a significant role in each of these important areas. Let's take a look at obesity first.

Increased obesity

One of the most pervasive risk factors for all major illnesses is obesity. Research has identified obesity as a risk factor in seven of the top 10 causes of death in the United States (see chart on page 132)—heart disease, cancer, stroke, respiratory diseases, diabetes, and Alzheimer's disease (more broadly speaking, dementia).

The body mass index (BMI) is used to determine if a person is overweight. The index identifies the ratio of weight to height but it does not provide information as to distribution of fat in the body. In addition to the BMI number, individuals are encouraged to evaluate the distribution of fat in their body. For example, studies indicate that excess fat around the midsection can be linked to cancer and heart disease. The combination of a high BMI and a larger waist circumference has been shown to be a dangerous risk factor for the development of serious illness. For more information about evaluating your risk as it relates to your weight, visit this website: http://www.nhlbi.nih.gov/health/public/heart/obesity/lose_wt/risk.htm.

According to the *UC Berkeley Wellness Letter* (June 2008), the "apple-shaped" body is associated with an increased risk of high blood pressure, several types of cancer, and dementia. "Since abdominal obesity often goes along with other factors that can increase dementia risk—such as diabetes, hypertension, and lack of physical activity—it is hard to know which is the main culprit," explain the UC Berkeley authors.

Body Mass Index (BMI) Chart

BMI (kg/m²)	19	20	21	22	23	24	25	26	27	28	29	30	35	40
Height (in.)	Weight (lb.)													
58	91	96	100	105	110	115	119	124	129	134	138	143	167	191
59	94	99	104	109	114	119	124	128	133	138	143	148	173	198
60	97	102	107	112	118	123	128	133	138	143	148	153	179	204
61	100	106	111	116	122	127	132	137	143	148	153	158	185	211
62	104	109	115	120	126	131	136	142	147	153	158	164	191	218
63	107	113	118	124	130	135	141	146	152	158	163	169	197	225
64	110	116	122	128	134	140	145	151	157	163	169	174	204	232
65	114	120	126	132	138	144	150	156	162	168	174	180	210	240
66	118	124	130	136	142	148	155	161	167	173	179	186	216	247
67	121	127	134	140	146	153	159	166	172	178	185	191	223	255
68	125	131	138	144	151	158	164	171	177	184	190	197	230	262
69	128	135	142	149	155	162	169	176	182	189	196	203	236	270
70	132	139	146	153	160	167	174	181	188	195	202	207	243	278
71	136	143	150	157	165	172	179	186	193	200	208	215	250	286
72	140	147	154	162	169	177	184	191	199	206	213	221	258	294
73	144	151	159	166	174	182	189	197	204	212	219	227	265	302
74	148	155	163	171	179	186	194	202	210	218	225	233	272	311
75	152	160	168	176	184	192	200	208	216	224	232	240	279	319
76	156	164	172	180	189	197	205	213	221	230	238	246	287	328

In 2008, researchers published their data evaluating more than 44,000 women involved in the Nurses' Health Study. They found that abdominal obesity was "strongly and positively associated with all-cause cardiovascular disease and cancer mortality." The researchers found that, even in women with a normal BMI, a large waist circumference was associated with an increased risk of heart disease.

Researchers from the American Cancer Society demonstrated that, among 95,151 study participants, a larger waist circumference was associated with an increased risk of colon cancer. They also showed that this risk was "partially independent of BMI." Other studies have shown a link between abdominal obesity and cancers of the breast, pancreas, and uterus.

Several studies have demonstrated that waist circumference is a better predictor of diabetes than BMI. A 2007 study involving nearly

Leading Causes of Death in the U.S.	Approximate %
1. Heart Disease	27
2. Cancer	23
3. Stroke	6
4. Respiratory Diseases (COPD and Asthma)	5
5. Accidents	5
6. Diabetes	3
7. Alzheimer's Disease	3
8. Influenza and Pneumonia	3
9. Kidney Disease	2
10. Septicemia (blood infection)	1

Source: Center for Disease Control and Prevention 2005

Probiotics Enhance Gut Immunity

A significant portion of our immune system is in the digestive tract. Technically this is called gut-association lymphoid tissue or GALT. You can find GALT in the esophagus, tonsils, adenoids, intestine, and stomach. There is a close interaction between GALT and immune response. Several studies have shown that probiotics enhance immunity by stimulating GALT. Some demonstrate that probiotics specifically stimulate our innate immunity—the immune defenses we were born with. In addition, probiotics can protect the immunologic mucosal barrier within the digestive system. By doing this, probiotics also help alleviate inflammation. Further research is needed to determine if some probiotics actually stimulate specific immune cells or if their action creates more of a protective and systemic response.

6,000 adults conducted by researchers from Queen's University in Ontario, Canada, found that waist circumference was a valid predictor of diabetes and recommended it be added as a routine measure for identification of high-risk patients.

Interesting new research from Finland has shown that probiotics may help women lose belly fat, also known as central obesity, after pregnancy. The researchers randomly divided 256 women into three groups during their first trimester. At the end of the study, central obesity was found in 18 percent fewer women in the probiotic group compared to the group receiving a placebo (fake pill). Studying pregnant women allow researchers to not only gauge the effects of obesity on the mothers but also the children. According to researcher Kirsi Laitinen from the University of Turku in Finland, "Based on previous experiments, we hypothesize that the maternal diet may influence both glucose metabolism and weight in the children."

Obesity plays such a significant role in health and disease progression because it negatively affects three key body functions:

immunity, inflammation, and insulin resistance. A significant way to reduce obesity is with consistent physical activity (refer to the side bar on page 125).

Controlling insulin resistance

Insulin resistance, also known as glucose intolerance, is complicated. For the purpose of this discussion, we'll provide a quick overview on how insulin resistance can lead to illness.

Glucose is the primary energy source for all cells. Glucose circulates in the blood stream so it's there when we need it. The pancreas releases two hormones that help keep our blood sugar levels balanced. If we skip a meal, our blood sugar drops so the pancreas then releases glucogon, which signals the liver to convert glycogen to glucose. When we eat a meal—regardless of its contents—our blood sugar rises, which causes the pancreas to release insulin. Insulin and glucogon work together to keep blood glucose balanced. When blood sugar is out of balance, a variety of symptoms, and eventually illness, will develop.

This all too commonly occurs because the typical American consumes too much sugar and refined carbohydrates. This causes a constant flooding of glucose into the blood stream. As blood sugar levels are constantly elevated, cells and tissues become resistant to the insulin released by the pancreas. This is insulin resistance, which is a contribuor to syndrome X. After a prolonged period of increased insulin secretion, the pancreas can't keep up. As insulin levels then decrease because the pancreas can't maintain a state of high insulin output, blood sugar levels continue to increase. High blood sugar levels can lead to diabetes, eye problems, kidney failure, heart conditions, and cancer.

It is believed that probiotics can help breakdown large sugar molecules into smaller, more digestible molecules. Many studies have shown that probiotics can help control insulin resistance. A 2008 study

Probiotics for Kids

The scientific literature is clear that children can benefit from probiotics. Specific research involves antibiotic-induced diarrhea, eczema, dermatitis, and inflammatory bowel diseases. "The use of probiotics in diarrheal diseases of children is increasing," according to Stephen Guandalini, MD, of the University of Chicago. "Probiotics…have been tried in many double-blinded, randomized, placebo-controlled studies, and several well-conducted meta-analyses are now available."

A 2007 literature review of seven different studies involving 432 infants at high risk of developing eczema showed that there was a significant reduction in this condition in those who had prebiotics added to their milk or formula. Mothers who are pregnant may want to consider consuming probiotics and prebiotics during the last weeks of pregnancy and while breastfeeding.

Eczema can be one of the first signs of allergy during early childhood development. It is believed this is due to a weakened immune system that has not fully developed yet. According to the American Academy of Dermatologists, while 10 to 20 percent of all infants develop eczema, nearly half of those will grow out of it between the ages of five and 15. A 2009 study published in the *European Journal of Allergy and Clinical Immunology*, demonstrated that parental-reported eczema was nearly 60 percent lower in the group of infants taking a probiotic mixture compared to placebo during the first three months of life.

Researchers from Albert Einstein College of Medicine conclude, "The gastrointestinal flora plays a complex and important role in the development of healthy immunologic and digestive function in children." Probiotics are safe for children.

published in the *British Journal of Nutrition* showed that probiotics helped balance glucose metabolism of pregnant women. The effects extended over the 12-month postpartum period as well.

Several animal studies have shown probiotics to be effective at preventing diabetes. In a 2008 study featured in the *European*

Journal of Drug Metabolism and Pharmacokinetics, researchers found that probiotics, combined with the anti-diabetes drug gliclazide (Glipizide), improved the bioavailability of the drug. The researchers concluded that probiotics may be beneficial as a complementary treatment for individuals with diabetes. Human clinical trials are needed to confirm the treatment effects of probiotics in cases of diabetes.

Keep in mind, type 1 and type 2 diabetes are serious medical conditions that requires close supervision from a qualified healthcare expert. Never discontinue taking a prescription medication without first discussing it with your doctor. Also be sure to inform your doctor of all of the dietary supplements you are taking. For more information about diabetes, refer to the next chapter.

One of the ways insulin resistance influences illness is by weakening the immune system. The two often go hand-in-hand.

Decreased immunity

The immune system is our first-line of defense against foreign invaders. There are trillions of specialized cells in the immune system that identify, capture, and then kill harmful cells. These cells circulate throughout our lymphatic system, stopping along the way to fight our internal battles against infection and disease. Immune cells gather in lymph nodes that are strategically placed throughout the body.

The immune system is very complex and we are only now just scratching the surface as to its role in health and disease. We do know that free radicals—highly reactive molecules that can damage healthy cells—can take a toll on our immune system. We kill free radicals with antioxidants. But when our antioxidant stores are depleted, the immune system becomes deficient and can't counter the damage to our cells, tissues, and organs. Antioxidant foods and dietary supplements are critical to the health of our immune system. Good bacteria have also been shown to directly scavenge free radicals. These bacteria

Mental Health Medicine

So far we've learned a lot about bad bugs. We know that bad bacteria and bacterial imbalance can make us very sick. But can bad bugs make us crazy? For many years we have known that, if left untreated, microbes such as *treponema pallidum* and *streptococcus* can lead to psychiatric disorders. This idea was explored back in the 1800s but, as soon as Freudian psychotherapy became popular, this notion was forgotten. That is, until recently. Scientists now believe there is strong evidence to suggest that schizophrenia, bipolar disorder, and obsessive-compulsive disorder can be linked to bacterial infections.

Researchers from Bristol University have even taken this one step further by contending that not only can bad bacteria cause mental illness, good bacteria may be able to alleviate it. Their work focused on clinical depression and was the result of outcomes involving cancer patients. An oncologist at the Royal Marsden Hospital in London found that when she gave her lung cancer patients an experimental treatment, they experienced an improvement in their emotional health as well. The experimental treatment was a bacteria known as *Mycobacterium vaccae*, a relative of tuberculosis.

Researchers at Johns Hopkins continue to explore this area of research. They are convinced they will find that infectious bacteria can lead to schizophrenia and bipolar disorder in certain susceptible individuals.

Related research from the Integrative Care Centre of Toronto, Canada, has shown that probiotics can help ease the emotional anxiety associated with chronic fatigue syndrome. Researchers involved with this randomized, double-blind, placebo-controlled human clinical trial concluded, "These results lend further support to the presence of a gut-brain interface, one that may be mediated by microbes that reside or pass through the intestinal tract."

have significant antioxidant activity. In addition to probiotics, here is a short list of where important antioxidants may be found:

- citrus fruits
- dark berries, specifically pomegranate and açai
- cocoa
- colorful vegetables
- green tea
- garlic
- oregano, curcumin, ginger, and rosemary

Nutrient-deficiencies, especially of important antioxidants such as vitamins A, C, D, and E, as well as zinc and selenium, can lead to a weakened immune system. A weakened immune system can be linked to numerous illnesses such as chronic fatigue syndrome, cancer, and many others. We all have circulating cancer cells in our body. The reason we don't all develop cancer is, in part, due to the strength of our immune system's ability to search out and destroy those cancer cells.

The immune system is set up to recognize self and non-self. But, when the cells fail to make this distinction, autoimmune conditions can develop. This occurs when the cells of the immune system attack healthy cells by mistake. Autoimmune disorders result from an overactive immune response. Examples of autoimmune conditions include allergy, multiple sclerosis, rheumatoid arthritis, lupus, thyroid disease, and celiac. The cause of autoimmune diseases is unknown, but there is an inherited predisposition in most cases (e.g., a family history). Often, this overzealous and inappropriate immune response comes from our inflammatory system. We'll discuss inflammation in more detail in the next section.

In addition to consuming more antioxidants through diet and dietary supplements, you can stimulate your immune system by doing the following:

- reduce consumption of sugar and simple carbohydrates
- reduce or eliminate alcohol

- don't smoke
- stay hydrated
- take a probiotic supplement daily
- exercise daily
- get enough sleep

There is a direct connection between the gastrointestinal tract and our immune system. As mentioned previously, the majority (about 70 percent) of our immune system resides in the digestive tract. This is often referred to as gut-associated lymphoid tissue (GALT). For more information refer to the side bar on page 133.

Several studies show that probiotics can positively influence many aspects of our immune system. A double-blind study featured in the March 2009 issue of the *British Journal of Nutrition* demonstrated that a symbiotic (a probiotic and a prebiotic combined) improved gut immune markers in people over age 65 who use non-steroidal anti-inflammatory drugs (NSAIDs). This is significant because long term NSAID use is associated with ulcers and decreased immunity.

In 2009, Dutch researchers reported that a possible immune enhancing effect of probiotics could be their activation of specific genes in the intestinal wall that helps establish immune tolerance. Their preliminary studies were presented at the Proceedings of the National Academy of Sciences.

Scientists at the Institute of Food Research published their human study in the journal *Clinical and Experimental Allergy*, demonstrating that *Lactobacillus casei* helped individuals suffering with hay fever symptoms. In 2009, the Chinese Department of Health approved anti-allergy claims for probiotic products.

A small study featured in the *Journal of Hepatology* showed an improvement in the immune function of white blood cells of alcoholics. *Lactobacillus fermentum* was shown to boost immune health in long distance runners according to research published in the *British Journal of Sports Medicine*.

Another body function that the immune system is intimately associated with is the inflammatory response. Controlling inflammation is critical to controlling serious illness.

Increased inflammation

Our reaction to an injury is inflammation. This is the immune system's way of healing the injury. Blood vessels dilate and white blood cells are sent to the scene. Neutrophils (particularly NK or natural killer cells) are a type of white blood cell that removes foreign particles in the area. Other cells are sent to help resolve the situation. This inflammatory response initially can cause swelling, bruising, redness, and pain, but eventually the injury is resolved.

Even if we don't have a readily recognized injury, internally our bodies respond with the same type of inflammatory response. First, there is a trigger such as a bacteria, virus, or oxidative tissue damage. Then the immune system springs into action with its inflammatory healing response. However, there are a variety of circumstances that can lead to a chronic, unrelenting inflammatory response including:

- too many free radicals and not enough antioxidants
- poor diet and nutrient deficiency
- chronic stress
- insulin resistance
- weakened immunity
- obesity

You can see how these factors all tie together. Chronic internal inflammation has been linked to a variety of illnesses, including all of the serious ones previously mentioned: cancer, heart disease, and diabetes.

An interesting study from 2009, published in the journal *Alcohol* evaluated intestinal inflammation and gut permeability of alcoholics. According to the researchers, "Because only 30 percent of alcoholics develop alcoholic liver disease, a factor other than heavy alcohol consumption must be involved in the development of alcohol-induced liver injury." They found that beneficial bacteria significantly reduced inflammation in both the intestine and liver, and also reduced gut permeability.

It's not surprising that the same ways you stimulate immunity will also help control chronic inflammation. Reducing internal inflammation is possible through a healthful diet, lifestyle, and dietary supplements.

10

SPECIFIC CONDITIONS

AS WE HAVE LEARNED, a whole host of problems can arise either through a leaky gut or when bad bacteria outnumber good bacteria— or through a combination of each. Because of this, most common illnesses can be directly or indirectly linked to bacterial issues.

All of the conditions profiled in the remainder of this chapter will benefit from the bacterial balance plan featured in the next section. Because we feel that taking a probiotic supplement daily will help ease these conditions, we did not list it in the treatment section of every condition. In some cases, however, we chose to highlight some of the newer scientific information involving probiotics for that particular condition. For most people, especially those suffering from one or more conditions featured in this chapter, a probiotic supplement should be taken just as you would a daily multi-vitamin/mineral supplement.

Please keep in mind that the following information on these specific conditions is not intended to be comprehensive. These are overviews to provide you with general knowledge about each condition. If you feel you have one of these conditions, discuss your concerns with your physician. Proper diagnosis is vital and we do not advocate self-diagnosis or self-treatment.

Acne

Description And Causes

Acne is one of the most common skin disorders in the world. According to the Acne Resource, 85 percent of people, age 12 to 24, have acne. But, acne is not just common among teens. Anyone can have acne, regardless of age or ethnicity. The American Dermatologist Association reports that 60 million American have active acne.

Acne is caused by three key factors:

- the *bacteria propionium*
- excess oil production
- poor exfoliation

In addition, hormonal changes such as those during the teen years or pregnancy, and diet can contribute to acne. Acne is characterized by blackheads, whiteheads, pustules, and/or cysts.

Treatment

Conventional treatment of acne can include topical over-the-counter and prescription medications, as well as physical procedures such as chemical peels and surgical extraction. These conventional treatments are not without their side effects and, in some cases, can worsen acne. We recommend trying a more natural approach first.

When dealing with acne, it's very important to use nontoxic products. Natural products will be gentler on your skin. Gentle, consistent exfoliation, cleansing, and hydration are all important to successfully treating acne.

For more information about acne, and skin care in general, refer to *Return To Beautiful Skin* by Myra Michelle Eby and Karolyn A. Gazella (Basic Health 2008). We recommend MyChelle Dermaceuticals, a natural skin care company that makes products which are always free of parabens, phthalates, propylene glycol, ureas, EDTA, and other toxic compounds commonly found in many skin care products (for more information visit www.mychelleusa.com). In addition, Essential Formulas Incorporated has an entire line of probiotic skin care treatments. For more information, visit www.essentialformulas.com. In addition to probiotics supplements, probiotics skin care products can help relieve acne.

Allergy

Description And Causes

Allergies occur when the immune system overreacts to an allergen. An allergen can come from food or from the environment. Allergies are considered autoimmune conditions because they are the result of an overactive immune response. For example, if your immune system views pollen, animal dander, or wheat as a dangerous invader, it will react by stimulating an inflammatory response.

When an allergen is removed—for example when the pollen season ends—the immune system stops reacting and the body returns to normal. If the allergen is never removed, the immune system stays on high alert, which can cause all types of symptoms and health issues.

Just as varied as the types of allergies are the causes. In some cases, we don't know exactly what causes allergies. We do know that certain circumstances can contribute to the development of allergies and/or the severity of symptoms including:

- diet (specifically a diet that creates nutritional deficiencies)
- depressed immune system
- stress
- genetics
- poor digestion, elimination, and detoxification

Typical symptoms of allergy include nasal congestion, sneezing, watery eyes, rashes, headache, fatigue, and swelling of the throat and tongue.

Treatment

Conventional allergy medications include antihistamines, decongestants, nasal sprays, steroids, and others. Allergy shots are used to desensitize the system. Most studies show that these shots are effective for inhaled allergies associated with pollens, molds, dust mites, and pet dander. Allergy shots have not been shown to be effective for eczema, hives, food allergies, or stinging-insect sensitivity.

The treatment of allergy depends on the type of allergy. For example, if it is a food allergy, you will want to identify and eliminate the offending food. Nearly all allergies will benefit from anti-inflammatory, immune-enhancing approach. Many studies have demonstrated that probiotics can help ease many different types of allergies.

Dietary supplements to consider include:

- **vitamin C** = 1,000 mg 3x daily
- **vitamin A** = 10,000 IU 3x daily
- **vitamin B12** = 1,000 mcg per day in the morning on an empty stomach
- **pantethine** = 300 mg 3x daily
- **quercetin** = 1,000 mg 3x daily with meals
- **magnesium** = 500 mg 3x daily with meals
- **Active Hexose Correlated Compound (AHCC)** = 500 mg per day with a meal
- **fish oils** = 1,000 mg 3x daily with meals
  NOTE: A quality vegetarian alternative to fish oils is Dr. Ohhira's Essential Living Oils.
- **vitamin E** = 400 IU 2x daily
- **selenium** = 50 mcg 2x daily

People suffering from allergies (even those allergies not created by food) need to pay special attention to the diet. The most important dietary advice is to avoid sugar and simple carbohydrates.

For more information on successful treatment of allergy, refer to Dr. Pescatore's book, *The Allergy & Asthma Cure* (Wiley, 2003).

Arthritis

Description And Causes

Arthritis involves pain and inflammation of the joints. According to the CDC, it is the most common cause of disability in the United States. There are two main types of arthritis: osteoarthritis and rheumatoid arthritis. Rheumatoid arthritis is an autoimmune condition where the immune system attacks healthy joint cells. Osteoarthritis is a degenerative joint disease where the cartilage that cushions the joints wears down and bone is rubbing on bone. This is typically most common in the joints of the knees, hands, hips, and spine.

Symptoms of osteoarthritis include morning stiffness, restricted range of motion, and painful and swollen joints. In addition to these symptoms, individuals with rheumatoid arthritis may also experience deformed joints, fatigue, weakness, and chronic infections.

Treatment

Rheumatoid arthritis is typically controlled with very serious and potentially dangerous prescription drugs. With osteoarthritis, pharmaceuticals may be used as well. In severe cases, the joint can be replaced via surgery. People with arthritis often turn to nonsteroidal anti-inflammatory drugs (NSAIDs). Unfortunately, although these drugs can provide short-term relief, they have actually been shown to contribute to joint damage. A class of drugs known as COX-2 inhibitors may accelerate joint damage in the long run and may increase your risk of heart attack.

That's why we like to recommend some natural, nontoxic therapies to try first. Massage, acupuncture, hydrotherapy, and reflexology have all been shown to provide pain relief for those with arthritis. Natural substances that can support healthy joints, specifically in cases of osteoarthritis, include glucosamine sulfate, chondroitin sulfate, S-adenosylmethionine (SAMe), methyl-sulfonyl-methane

(MSM), boswellia, curcumin, and Celadrin, a natural esterfied fatty acid. Celadrin is also available as a topical cream. In 2004, researchers from the University of California, Irvine, compared SAMe to Celebrex in a double-blind study involving 61 adults diagnosed with osteoarthritis of the knee. The researchers noted that while it took longer for SAMe to start working, at the end of the trial it was just as effective as Celebrex—without the potential side effects. The dosage used in this study and others is 1,200 mg daily.

Being physically active is important with arthritis. In addition, maintaining a healthy weight will help reduce pressure on the joints.

Cancer

Description And Causes

Cancer is not just one condition. It is an extremely complex disease with more than 200 variations. Cancer is characterized by uncontrolled growth of an abnormal cell or group of cells. Cancers can inhabit an organ or tissue and can circulate in blood or throughout our lymph system. The most common form of cancer is a solid tumor that can inhabit nearly any organ or part of the body. Statistics from 2008 from the American Cancer Institute indicate that nonmelanoma skin cancer is the most commonly diagnosed cancer. Lung cancer is next on the list.

There are many contributors to the development of cancer including:

- environment
- poor diet
- genetics
- alcohol
- tobacco use

Individuals with a family history have a higher likelihood of developing cancer, however, only five to 10 percent of all cancers are caused by genetics. A family history indicates a predisposition, not an inevitable diagnosis.

Treatment

Conventional cancer treatment includes three primary tools: drugs, surgery, and radiation. Chemotherapy agents are the most common type of drugs used to treat cancer. There are dozens of chemotherapy drugs currently being used to treat cancer. These drugs can be very toxic. Radiation is also not without side effects. For this reason, more and more people with cancer are turning to an integrative approach that features complementary medicines such as dietary supplements.

Engaging in a healthier diet and lifestyle is absolutely critical to the success of the cancer patient. There are numerous studies showing that probiotics can also help individuals with cancer.

Most of the probiotic/cancer research involves colon cancer. Researchers featured in the February 2007 issue of the *American Journal of Clinical Nutrition* concluded, "Several colorectal cancer biomarkers can be altered favorably by symbiotic intervention." Researchers featured in the journal *Cancer Biology and Therapy* stated, "Probiotics and prebiotics have the potential to impact significantly on the development, progression, and treatment of colorectal cancer and may have a valuable role in cancer prevention." As mentioned in the previous chapter, the bacteria *H pylori* has been shown to cause stomach cancer.

Cancer treatment is extremely complex. For more information about integrative cancer treatment refer to the *Definitive Guide to Cancer* by Lise Alschuler, ND, and Karolyn A. Gazella (Celestial Arts, 2007, revised paperback edition 2010).

Celiac

Description And Causes

According to the University of Chicago Comer Children's Hospital, the prevalence of celiac disease in the United States is estimated to be as high as one in 133; however, only one in 4,700 individuals have been diagnosed with it. "The average delay in diagnosis for a person with symptoms is 11 years," reports the Comer Children's Hospital. "On average, a child will visit eight pediatricians before being diagnosed with celiac disease."

Celiac is an autoimmune response to gluten in the diet. If an individual with celiac eats gluten, which is a protein in wheat, rye, oats, spelt, and barley, his/her immune system will respond by attacking the small intestine. This causes a wide range of symptoms associated with digestive disturbance, including diarrhea, gas, constipation, abdominal pain, or bloating. Individuals with celiac can also experience depression, irritability, and fuzzy thinking.

We don't know exactly what causes celiac, but we do know that there can be a genetic factor. If you have a primary relative (parent or sibling) with celiac, you may have a predisposition to it as well. It is good to note that conventional medical wisdom believes that you either have celiac or you don't. We are now starting to understand that there is a spectrum of celiac or gluten sensitivity. You don't have to be a true celiac with the genetic marker to suffer from gluten/gliadin or wheat family sensitivities. It is important to have your blood tested in several different ways.

Treatment

The only known treatment for celiac disease is lifelong elimination of gluten—a gluten-free diet. Keep in mind, there is a spectrum of gluten sensitivity. Mild sensitivities with the ability to eat some wheat is on one end of the spectrum while celiac disease and the inability to eat any wheat is on the other end.

The Celiac Sprue Association warns, "While one would expect to find gluten in places like breads, pastas, cookies, and other obvious grain products, gluten is also 'hidden' in many processed foods such as frozen French fried potatoes, soy sauce, and rice cereal." Most natural health stores have a wide range of gluten-free products to choose from. For a complete list of foods that contain gluten, you may visit www.livingwithout.com.

In addition to probiotics, there is a product called Gluten Defense by Enzymatic Therapy that includes gluten-digesting enzymes. This product is not intended to "cure" celiac disease. However, it can help individuals tolerate small amounts of hidden gluten in foods. Keep in mind, taking dietary supplements is not recommended as a treatment for celiac disease. The only effective treatment is the avoidance of gluten.

Colitis

Description and Causes

This condition is characterized by ulcers in the lining of the colon and rectum. It is classified as an inflammatory bowel disease. This condition is typically diagnosed in individuals age 15 to 30 and it tends to run in families. It is a life-long condition.

Common symptoms of colitis include abdominal pain, bloody diarrhea, and/or an unexplained fever that last more than a day or two. Individuals with colitis could also experience anemia, severe fatigue, weight loss, loss of appetite, skin sores, and joint pain. It is estimated that about 50 percent of individuals with colitis have only mild symptoms. In severe cases, a surgical removal of the colon may be necessary. Although colitis is not considered a fatal disease, it can cause life-threatening complications.

Treatment

There is no cure for colitis. Conventional medicine uses drugs to manage symptoms. Some of the drugs have side effects such as nausea, headache, a worsening of diarrhea, insomnia, allergic reactions, and kidney and liver damage. According to the May 2006 issue of the *Journal of the American Medical Association*, the drug Remicade increases the risk of developing several types of cancer including lymphoma, skin, gastrointestinal, breast, and lung.

The treatment goal with colitis is to ease inflammation. For this reason, an anti-inflammatory diet and dietary supplements with anti-inflammatory properties are effective. Fresh whole foods, especially colorful fruits and vegetables, are anti-inflammatory. Herbs that have anti-inflammatory properties include curcumin and boswellia. Essential fatty acids also are anti-inflammatory. Taking a quality probiotic on an ongoing basis has a tendency to ease the number and severity of colitis attacks.

Crohn's Disease

Description And Causes

Crohn's disease is an inflammatory bowel disease that can affect any and all areas along the entire digestive system. It most commonly affects the lower part of the small intestine. Although it is most often diagnosed in young adults, Crohn's can occur at any age. There can be a genetic predisposition in some cases.

Symptoms of Crohn's include abdominal pain, diarrhea, rectal bleeding, fever, skin problems, weight loss, intestinal blockage, fatigue, and malnutrition. Symptoms of Crohn's can vary dramatically from one individual to the next and they can change over time. In severe cases, symptoms are not limited to the digestive system and can include joint pain, eye problems, and issues with the skin and liver. Children with Crohn's disease may experience delayed growth.

Crohn's disease can be hard to diagnose because there is no single test that conclusively points to Crohn's. A combination of information including patient history, symptoms, physical exam, x-rays, and pathology reports are used to diagnose Crohn's.

Treatment

There is no cure for Crohn's. Drugs are used to suppress the inflammatory response and surgery is often indicated at some point. Surgery is used to remove diseased segments, repair damage, or eliminate blockages.

Proper nutrition is critical with Crohn's. This condition is associated with poor absorption of nutrients, as well as dietary protein, fat, carbohydrates, and water. This can rob the body of important fluids, as well as vitamins and minerals. According to the Crohn's & Colitis Foundation of America, when Crohn's is active, soft, bland foods may cause less discomfort than spicy and high-fiber foods. Keep in mind, however, that the diet does not cause Crohn's but it can help reduce symptoms and promote healing.

Using a natural approach that includes an anti-inflammatory diet and dietary supplements as described in the colitis section may help individuals with Crohn's. Several studies evaluating the effectiveness of essential fatty acids involving patients with Crohn's have had positive outcomes including improved remission rates and fewer relapses. Individuals with Crohn's have been shown to be deficient in most of the key vitamins and minerals. The only exception is copper. Copper levels are often elevated and should be avoided. Preliminary research and isolated case studies have demonstrated that probiotics can help improve the quality of life and reduce new episodes in some Crohn's patients.

Dementia

Description And Causes

Dementia is actually not a disease, it is a symptom caused by disorders that affect brain function. Individuals with dementia may have two or more of these symptoms:

- memory loss
- confusion
- language difficulties
- loss of problem-solving ability
- inability to control emotions
- inability to do simple tasks such as eating or getting dressed
- personality changes
- behavioral issues
- delusions or hallucinations

Some of the diseases that can cause dementia include Alzheimer's disease, Parkinson's disease, Huntington's disease, and vascular dementia (strokes). Dementia is not a normal part of aging.

Treatment

Presently, there is no cure for many of the disease causes of dementia. Pharmaceutical agents are used to slow progression and control symptoms. Prevention and early diagnosis are critical.

Natural substances shown to improve brain function include gingko biloba, citicholine, phosphatidylserine and a special extract from Lion's mane mushrooms. Japanese researchers have shown that Lion's mane extract inhibited the formation of toxic peptides in brain cells and stimulated nerve growth factor in the brain. More research on these substances is needed to determine their effectiveness in slowing the progression of dementia and Alzheimer's.

New research featured in the journal *Neurobiology of Aging* demonstrated that being physically active can also help improve blood flow to the brain. "Being sedentary is now considered a risk factor for stroke and dementia," said study author Marc Poulin, an associate professor at the University of Calgary. "Our findings also show that better blood flow translates into improved cognition."

Diabetes

Description And Causes

About 21 million Americans have been diagnosed with diabetes, and it is estimated that an additional 20 million don't know they have it. These individuals are likely to have the most common form of diabetes known as type 2. In fact, more than two-thirds of those with diabetes have this form of the disease. Type 2 diabetes is on the rise primarily due to the increase in obesity, a key risk factor for diabetes. Type 2 diabetes was previously referred to as adult-onset diabetes because it only affected adults. Today, however, the standard American diet (SAD) has caused many children to develop this form of diabetes, putting them at risk of developing serious illnesses later in life or struggling with serious side effects of the condition.

Diabetes occurs when blood sugar levels are too high. As mentioned in the last chapter, two hormones help us control blood sugar levels: glucogon and insulin. Type 1 diabetes is diagnosed in children, teenagers, and young adults. It is an autoimmune condition where the pancreas no longer makes insulin because the body's immune system has attacked and destroyed the cells needed to make the hormone. Type 1 diabetes is not caused by diet, however symptoms can be exacerbated by a diet high in sugar.

With type 2 diabetes, the body does not use insulin properly and the pancreas eventually stops secreting the insulin needed. This form of diabetes begins with insulin resistance (refer to Chapter 9 for more information). Some individuals can also have pre-diabetes, which occurs when blood sugar levels are higher than normal but not high enough to warrant a diabetes diagnosis. It is estimated that many people with pre-diabetes will develop type 2 diabetes within ten years. Weight loss and exercise have been shown to reverse pre-diabetes or delay a type 2 diagnosis.

Symptoms of diabetes can vary from one individual to the next. According to the American Diabetes Association, here is a list of common symptoms:

- frequent urination
- excessive thirst
- extreme hunger
- unusual weight loss
- increased fatigue
- irritability
- blurry vision

There are three different tests to diagnose diabetes including fasting plasma glucose, oral glucose tolerance, glycosalated hemoglobin and random plasma glucose. If you feel you may have diabetes, talk to your doctor.

Treatment

Individuals with type 1 diabetes must monitor their insulin levels very carefully and must be under the careful care of a healthcare professional. Healthful food choices are the foundation of treatment for anyone with diabetes. This includes:

- limiting or eliminating alcohol intake
- limiting sweets and dramatically reducing sugar intake
- eating frequently
- limiting the amount of simple carbohydrates

For type 2 diabetes, many nutritional supplements have been shown to help stabilize glucose levels by improving the efficiency of insulin so more glucose is burned for energy rather than stored as fat. In 2006, Yale University researchers demonstrated that chromium picolinate combined with biotin helps control glucose in individuals with type 2 diabetes. The daily dosage is 600 mg of chromium and 2 mg biotin. Other natural substances that have been shown to help control blood sugar levels include cinnamon, gymnemma sylvestre, and green tea. The antioxidant alpha-lipoic acid has been found to help reduce complications of diabetes, specifically nerve damage or peripheral neuropathy. A dosage of 100 mg of pycnogenol has also been shown in clinical studies to be effective.

As mentioned previously, probiotics help prevent and treat diabetes by easing inflammation, enhancing immunity, and reducing insulin resistance.

If you have type 1 diabetes, discuss all natural options and dietary supplements with your doctor. Never discontinue taking medications without your doctor's approval.

Diarrhea

Description And Causes

If you have loose, watery stools more than three times in one day, you have diarrhea. Diarrhea can also cause cramps, nausea, and bloating. Diarrhea is considered a symptom rather than a disease. It is not usually life-threatening, but it can indicate a more serious problem such as colon cancer, inflammatory bowel disease, or some other digestive illness. If diarrhea persists for more than three days and you are dehydrated, see your doctor. Keep in mind, diarrhea can be more dangerous in children so seek medical care if your child has diarrhea for several days in a row.

There are a variety of potential causes of diarrhea including bacteria, viruses, parasites, food intolerances, some medication, and gastrointestinal diseases. In some cases, no direct cause can be identified. Travelers sometimes experience diarrhea. For more information refer to the section on traveler's diarrhea. Antibiotic use can also cause diarrhea. This can be especially harmful in children.

Treatment

Most cases of diarrhea will resolve without treatment. There are several over-the-counter (OTC) medications available to help relieve diarrhea; however, keep in mind that diarrhea will last as long with or without these medications. These OTC drugs are designed to help with symptom relief. One side effect of loperamide (Imodium) is that it can cause constipation. Bismuth subsalicylates (Pepto-Bismol, Kaopectate) can cause your tongue and stool to turn dark, which is a short-term side effect.

Probiotics are by far the best natural treatment for diarrhea. Several clinical studies have confirmed that probiotics will help heal antibiotic-induced diarrhea in both children and adults.

Too much vitamin C or magnesium can often cause diarrhea and should be avoided if you are experiencing diarrhea. If you have diarrhea, it is important to stay hydrated. Here are some other tips to try to help relieve diarrhea:

- eat brown rice and water
- avoid solid foods for the first 24 hours; eat soup broth instead
- stay away from spicy and rich foods
- avoid caffeine and carbonated drinks

Remember, diarrhea is not necessarily bad. It helps to rid your body of toxins. Be patient. It is likely that within a couple of days, you will be back to normal.

Diverticulitis

Description And Causes

A low-fiber diet may cause diverticulitis, which is the development of small pouches that bulge in the colon. This condition is more common in individuals over the age of 60. Most people with diverticulitis don't even know they have it because there are very few symptoms. Sometimes it can cause mild cramping, bloating, and constipation. If the pouches become inflamed and infected, a fever can develop. In some cases, diverticulitis can cause nausea, vomiting, chills, or cramping. In serious cases, blockages can develop.

Treatment

Antibiotics may be prescribed to clear up infections. Although a low-fiber diet causes this condition, it is a low-fiber diet that is indicated during flare-ups. After symptoms improve, high-fiber foods can be reintroduced to the diet. Recurrent attacks of diverticulitis can cause serious damage to the colon. Surgery may be required to remove the damaged portion of the intestine. Probiotics are highly recommended for anyone who has been on antibiotics.

E Coli Infection

Description And Causes

Unfortunately, *E coli* contamination has become more common. *E coli* is a type of bacteria that lives in the intestines. Most types of this bacterium are harmless. Other types can cause traveler's diarrhea and even death. Children and adults with a weak immune system are most vulnerable to this bad bug.

E coli infections come from eating foods that contain the harmful bacteria. You can also get this infection by swallowing water in a swimming pool that contains *E coli*.

Symptoms of *E coli* infection can include severe stomach cramps, diarrhea that can be bloody, and vomiting. People of any age can get infected. Typically, the infection will get better in about five to seven days. Testing of a stool sample can determine if the infecting bacterium is *E coli*.

Treatment

Antibiotics should not be used for *E coli* infection. This can lead to antibiotic resistance and side effects. There is also no evidence to suggest that antibiotics are effective against *E coli* bacteria. The best treatment for *E coli* infection is to provide supportive care. Preventing dehydration is important. To stay properly hydrated, drink at least eight 8-ounce glasses of pure water daily and avoid dehydrating liquids like caffeinated drinks and alcohol.

To prevent *E coli* infection, be sure to wash hands thoroughly and frequently, cook meats thoroughly, avoid unpasteurized products, and avoid ingesting the water in pools, lakes, ponds, and streams.

Japanese researcher Ohhira has shown that his bacterial strain, TH10, is effective at battling *E coli* infection.

Eczema

Description And Causes

Eczema is a skin condition also known as dermatitis. Atopic dermatitis is the most common type of eczema. It is an allergic condition that causes the skin to become itchy and dry. It is commonly found in babies and young children. Eczema can also cause the skin to become red and swollen.

Several factors can cause eczema such as irritating substances in your skin care products, allergies, or other illnesses. Diet and lifestyle—specifically high levels of stress—can exacerbate symptoms and cause flare-ups. Eczema can run in families.

Treatment

Eczema cannot be cured, but it can successfully be controlled. Symptom relief is a key goal of eczema treatment. When itching and inflammation is severe or there is a skin infection, medications may be prescribed.

The best way to prevent eczema flare-ups is with a multi-pronged approach that includes diet, lifestyle, and dietary supplements. Avoid triggers in the diet such as dairy or wheat. Practice stress reduction techniques such as yoga, meditation, or deep breathing. Be sure to use only natural skin care products, especially when it comes to hydrating creams. In addition to probiotics, gamma-linolenic acid (GLA) from borage or evening primose oil has been shown to be effective in controlling eczema flare-ups. Topically, you can try virgin coconut oil and oatmeal baths. Just add a couple cups of rolled oats from the grocery store to your warm bath.

Try to avoid using topical steroid creams. Over time these creams can cause the skin to become thin. Probiotic skin care products may be an effective alternative.

Gastroenteritis (Stomach Flu)

Description And Causes

At some point, we all have experienced stomach flu. This is known as gastroenteritis. You can get gastroenteritis when you have contact with an infected person or ingest contaminated food or water. This viral condition causes diarrhea (non-bloody), abdominal cramps, nausea, vomiting, and sometimes fever. Some people may experience muscle aches or headaches.

Viral gastroenteritis will typically run its course and you will feel much better in 24 to 48 hours. This condition can, however, be deadly in infants, older adults, or individuals with a compromised immune system.

Adults should seek medical attention under the following circumstances:

- unable to keep liquids down for 24 hours
- vomiting for more than 48 hours
- vomiting blood
- experiencing signs of dehydration such as excessive thirst, dry mouth, little or no urine, or severe weakness
- there is blood in your bowel movements
- a fever of 104 degrees F or higher

Seek medical treatment for a child right away if these symptoms are exhibited:

- temperature of 102 degrees F or higher
- experiencing a lot of pain or discomfort
- bloody diarrhea
- seems dehydrated

In the case of an infant, call your doctor right away if the baby is vomiting for more than several hours, hasn't had a wet diaper in six hours, has bloody stools or severe diarrhea, cries without tears, or is unusually sleepy and unresponsive. Please remember that the above is simply a guideline and by no means should be used without the direction of your own personal physician. If you experience any of these symptoms, please contact your physician.

Treatment

Gastroenteritis is diagnosed based on symptoms. There is no specific medical treatment for this illness and antibiotics are not effective. The herb ginger has anti-nausea properties and may help to ease symptoms.

To avoid dehydration, drink plenty of fluids. Prevention is key with the stomach flu so be sure to wash hands thoroughly and avoid close contact with someone who has the virus. If you are susceptible, you may also want to take additional probiotics during cold and flu season.

Gastroesophageal Reflux Disease (GERD)

Description And Causes

There is a muscle at the end of your esophagus just before your stomach called the lower esophageal sphincter (LES). GERD occurs when this muscle does not close properly. Stomach juices, specifically acid, can then back up or reflux into the esophagus causing irritation. This is known as heartburn. When heartburn occurs more than two times a week, it is known as gastroesophageal reflux disease.

According to the American College of Gastroenterology, more than 60 million Americans experience heartburn at least once a month and about 15 million experience heartburn every day. Heartburn is also called acid indigestion and is more common in the elderly and in pregnant women.

When the esophagus is exposed to the harsh stomach juices for an extended period of time, it can damage the esophageal lining, which causes burning and discomfort. Most people describe GERD as a burning sensation that begins behind the breastbone and travels up towards the throat. Some will experience a bitter or sour taste in the back of their throat because of the acid. Heartburn associated with GERD can last for several hours and will usually get worse after eating.

If you experience heartburn more than twice a week, see your doctor. It could be a sign of a more serious condition. If left untreated, GERD can also lead to more severe problems including chest pain that mimics a heart attack, narrowing or obstruction of the esophagus, bleeding, or a pre-malignant change in the esophageal lining known as Barrett's esophagus. People with untreated GERD have a higher risk of developing esophageal cancer.

Treatment

A variety of OTC and prescription medications are available to treat GERD. These include antacids (e.g. Tums), H2 blockers (e.g. Pepcid), and proton pump inhibitors (e.g. Prilosec). Side effects of the overuse of antacids include constipation, diarrhea, and stomach cramps. Side effects of H2 blockers and proton pump inhibitors include confusion, chest tightness, sore throat, fever, weakness, headaches, dizziness, and diarrhea. Bear in mind that many Americans take these medications on a daily basis. We have no idea what the side effects of long-term usage are. It has never been clinically tested, so think twice before popping that little purple pill.

These medications are designed to block stomach acid. While it may be counter-intuitive, the best treatment for GERD may be the addition of natural digestive enzymes including betaine hydrochloric acid taken with meals. With some individuals, symptoms will subside when digestion is aided rather than simply blocking stomach acid production. Enteric-coated peppermint oil can also help with GERD. It's important that peppermint oil capsules are enteric-coated because then the oil will be able to get past the stomach and be delivered to the intestines.

From a diet and lifestyle standpoint, get to know the foods that trigger heartburn. This often includes alcohol, spicy, fatty, or acidic foods. Eat smaller meals and do not eat close to bedtime. For individuals who are carrying extra weight, weight loss will help reduce the symptoms of GERD.

To relieve the symptoms of GERD, we recommend chewing one capsule of Dr. Ohhira's Probiotic 12 PLUS prior to each meal.

For more information, refer to Martie Whittekin's book, *Natural Alternatives to Nexium, Maalox, Tagamet, Priolsec and Other Acid Blockers* (Square One Publishers, 2009).

Gingivitis (Gum Disease)

Description And Causes

Inflammation of the gums is known as gingivitis. Plaque is the buildup of film on the teeth. When that buildup becomes hardened and accumulates at the gum line, the gum tissue becomes inflamed.

Signs that you may have gingivitis include:

- puffy or swollen gums
- receding or painful gums
- bleeding when you brush your teeth
- loose teeth
- bad breath that does not go away and is unrelated to food

The number one cause of gingivitis is poor dental hygiene. Brushing and flossing helps keep plaque at bay. Teeth should be brushed at least twice a day and flossed at least once a day. Regular dental check-ups are also important.

Smoking also causes gum disease because there is decreased oxygen delivery to gum tissue. This makes it easier for bacteria to invade the gums. Poor nutrition and nutritional deficiencies can contribute to gum disease as well. Individuals with diabetes are also at a higher risk of developing gingivitis.

Treatment

The best way to treat gingivitis is to proactively prevent it. In severe cases, dental treatments may be recommended including gum surgery, bone grafts, or placement of antibiotics into the gum tissue.

Nan Fuchs, PhD, editor of the *Women's Health Letter*, has a unique way of treating gum disease. She takes one to two capsule of Dr. Ohhira's Probiotics 12 PLUS and holds them in the mouth until the capsule softens. She then bites them enough to squeeze out some of the probiotic paste at the base of the teeth around the gums. You can focus the paste on the painful and inflamed parts of the gum. Allow the paste to dissolve and swallow the rest. As it turns out, the advice Fuchs is delivering is now being scientifically validated. A 2007 report in the *Journal of Dental Research* confirmed the hypothesis that probiotics placed along the gum line will prevent the growth of the bad bacteria that causes gum disease. This is known as "guided pocket recolonization" and is an innovative approach to the treatment of gingivitis. Coenzyme Q10 (CoQ10) has also been shown to aid in the reduction of gum disease. Taking CoQ10 as a dietary supplement and also using an oral rinse that contains CoQ10 is an effective combination for gum health.

In addition to consistent brushing and flossing, don't smoke and reduce or eliminate simple sugars in your diet, especially high-sugar soda pop and candy.

Heart Disease

Description And Causes

Heart disease, also known as cardiovascular disease, is the number one killer in the world. Approximately 40 percent of all deaths in the United States can be attributed to heart disease. This is a broad topic and the term is used to describe a number of specific illnesses that affect blood vessels, problems associated with heart rhythm, and congenital heart defects. Heart disease refers to conditions that cause the blood vessels to become narrow or blocked. This can lead to a heart attack, angina (chest pain), or stroke.

Heart disease symptoms will vary among individuals and is dependent on the type of heart disease that is present. For example, men will likely have symptoms different from women. In general, here are the symptoms of heart disease:

- shortness of breath
- irregular heart beats, skipped beats, or a "flip-flop" feeling in the chest
- rapid heart rate
- weakness or dizziness
- nausea
- sweating

An actual heart attack can cause pain, pressure, or heaviness in the chest, arm, or below the breastbone. An individual may experience heartburn or discomfort that radiates to the back, jaw, throat, or arm. If you or someone you are with is having a heart attack, don't delay. Call 911 right away and then give them an aspirin.

Causes of heart disease may include:

- high blood pressure
- elevated cholesterol
- diabetes
- smoking

- excessive use of alcohol, caffeine, or drugs
- stress
- unhealthy diet
- lack of exercise
- obesity

Men are at higher risk of heart disease than women; however a woman's risk increases after menopause. Individuals with a family history are at higher risk, especially if a parent had heart disease at an early age.

Treatment

The treatment regimen for heart disease depends on the heart condition diagnosed. Surgery or prescription drugs may be necessary. Everyone with heart disease will benefit from certain lifestyle changes including:

- increase exercise based on your doctor's recommendation
- if you smoke, quit
- lose weight when indicated
- increase consumption of fresh vegetables
- reduce consumption of simple sugars

If you have high cholesterol or high blood pressure, it is important to bring those into normal range. Many dietary supplements have been shown to benefit both of these conditions, as well as provide overall improvement to heart health. This includes probiotics, aged garlic extract, flavonoids from citrus fruits, plant sterols, and coenzyme Q10.

Inflammatory Bowel Disease
(*see* Colitis and Crohn's)

Irritable Bowel Syndrome

Description And Causes

The contraction of the intestines is what helps move food through our colon. If the intestines squeeze too hard or not hard enough, it can cause discomfort. This condition is known as irritable bowel syndrome (IBS). While IBS is not life threatening and will not damage the intestines, it can be very uncomfortable. It is the most common disorder diagnosed by gastroenterologists, affecting twice as many women as men.

The cause of IBS is unknown, however, stress and diet can exacerbate symptoms, which can include:

- abdominal cramping
- bloating and gas
- diarrhea
- constipation
- alternating diarrhea and constipation

Most people diagnosed with IBS can control their symptoms with diet and stress management.

Treatment

In 2008, the FDA approved the drug Amitiza to be used in adult women who have IBS with constipation. However, side effects of this drug include nausea, diarrhea, abdominal pain, fainting, dry mouth, difficulty breathing, and heart palpitations. Instead of drugs, first-line treatment should be centered around diet and dietary supplements.

From a dietary standpoint, increasing fiber may assist with symptom relief, but be sure to drink enough water with that fiber or you will get constipated. Dairy and caffeine can make IBS worse. We recommend you keep a food diary to determine exactly which foods make your symptoms flare. After identifying the culprits, reduce or eliminate those foods. As for dietary supplements, there is an impressive amount of research involving probiotics.

There is a home test kit know as ALCAT that is very effective at determining food sensitivites. For more information ask your doctor or visit www.alcat.com.

According to the president of the World Gastroenterology Association, Emmanon Quigley, MD, probiotics represents "the threshold of a new era of research and therapy for this [IBS] common disorder." There are numerous studies demonstrating the effectiveness of probiotics for IBS.

In addition to probiotics, enteric-coated peppermint oil has been shown to be effective in relieving IBS symptoms. The enteric coating ensures the peppermint passes through the stomach to the intestines where it then relaxes intestinal contractions and calms the colon. Enzymes with meals may also help. Keep in mind that antacids and any sugar alcohols such as sorbitol or any sweetener that ends in -ol can cause diarrhea, so they should be avoided.

Liver Disease

Description And Causes

The liver is the largest and one of the most significant organs in the human body. It serves hundreds of functions including the detoxification of harmful substances. The liver also helps transform food into energy. It stores and releases specific vitamins, minerals, and other nutrients. The liver controls the production and elimination of cholesterol, too. Because of these diverse functions, when the liver is damaged, it significantly affects many areas of the body.

Liver diseases are more common in those who drink large amounts of alcohol or who have been diagnosed with the hepatitis virus. Other risk factors include malnutrition, parasites, toxic chemicals, and congestive heart failure. Mixing alcohol with some medications, specifically acetaminophen (Tylenol) and statin drugs, is especially toxic to the liver and can cause permanent damage.

There are two types of liver cancer, primary and secondary. Primary is when it originates in the liver and secondary is when it has spread to the liver from a different area in the body such as bone or breast. Primary liver cancer is not as common but is growing rapidly in the number of cases. Liver cancer can be hard to detect and many types of liver cancer tend to grow rapidly.

Symptoms of liver disease are usually silent but may include jaundice (yellowing of the skin, eyes, and dark urine), severe weakness and fatigue, abdominal pain and swelling, fever, nausea, and vomiting.

Treatment

Treatment varies depending on the type of liver disease. It could include steroid, antiviral, or immunosuppressive drugs, or it could be surgery. The liver has the amazing ability to regenerate itself, so a diseased portion of the liver can be removed and the remaining liver will function just fine. A portion of a healthy liver can also be dissected and transplanted into another person. Liver transplant is another treatment option in severe cases of liver damage.

There are several natural substances that support liver function and detoxification. Probiotics for liver disease presents a promising new application for these beneficial bacteria. In addition, the herbs dandelion and milk thistle (silymarin) have been the focus of several clinical studies. The Auyervedic product LiverCare (internationally known as Liv.52) has been studied in nearly 200 clinical studies worldwide. This product contains a proprietary herbal blend and is available in natural health stores. Several studies have shown that Active Hexose Correlated Compound (AHCC) as a nutritional supplement is effective treatment for some liver diseases.

Osteoporosis

Description And Causes

Osteoporosis is characterized by thin, weak bones. Anyone can get osteoporosis, however it is most common in older women. According to the National Institutes of Health, as many as 50 percent of all women—and 25 percent of all men over the age of 50—will break a bone due to osteoporosis. It is considered a silent disease because many people don't even realize they have it until they break a bone.

Risk factors for osteoporosis include:

- thin with a small frame
- present or past issues with anorexia
- cigarette smoking
- excessive alcohol use
- sedentary lifestyle (lack of physical activity)
- family history
- having low bone mass (osteopenia)
- surgically-induced menopause
- some medication such as corticosteroids and anticonvulsants
- getting older
- Caucasian and Asian women

If you have experienced a gradual change in height or posture, you may want to ask your doctor about getting a bone mineral density test (BMD). The BMD test is the best way to determine if you have experienced bone loss.

Treatment

Primary treatment of osteoporosis includes drugs known as bisphosphonates (Fosamax, Actonel, and Boniva). Hormone drugs such as raloxifene (Evista) are approved to treat osteoporosis, however, there are concerns about the development of cancer and heart disease, so these drugs are not prescribed as frequently as the bisphophonates. The biphosphonates, especially the injectables, lead to an increased risk for osteonecrosis of the jaw and can have many other side effects, so it behooves you to take good care of your bones before it's too late.

Prevention is key. A diet rich in green leafy vegetables and low in sugar will help protect bone health. Soft drinks containing phosphoric acid should be avoided because they can cause calcium depletion.

Calcium, magnesium, vitamin D3, and vitamin K2 are critical to bone health. Zinc and boron are also important. Individuals at high risk of developing osteoporosis should take a dietary supplement that contains these important bone-building nutrients.

Many studies have shown that probiotics and prebiotics can help protect bone health. In fact, studies by Dr. Ohhira have shown that the use of probiotics increases the successful uptake of bone-building nutrients that help improve bone density.

Prostate Disorders

Description And Causes

The prostate gland is a part of the male reproductive system. This gland, which is about the size of a walnut in a young man, helps make semen. The prostate is near the urethra, the tube that carries urine out of the bladder. This gland tends to grow bigger with age. This can cause numerous symptoms associated with urination. When the prostate is enlarged, and it is not due to cancer, it is known as benign prostatic hyperplasia (BPH), which is common in men over age 50.

Symptoms of BPH include dribbling after urination, the urge to urinate frequently especially at night, and less urine flow.

Another condition that can affect the prostate is prostatitis or inflammation due to a bacterial infection. Burning and pain during urination is a symptom of prostatitis, which usually affects younger men.

Having one prostate disorder does not increase your chances of having another. They are all separate and independent of each other. For example, if you have prostatitis, you are not at risk of developing BPH or prostate cancer.

Treatment

Conventional treatment of both BPH and prostatitis includes prescription medications. A popular and widely studied natural treatment for BPH is the herb saw palmetto. Several small studies and one large clinical trial completed in 2006 have confirmed that saw palmetto can help provide relief of symptoms associated with moderate to severe BPH.

Anti-inflammatory and anti-bacterial herbs such as curcumin, goldenseal, olive leaf extract and oregano may provide relief for men with prostatitis. A yeast-free diet, and the reduction of caffeine and spicy foods may also help.

If you feel you may have an issue with your prostate gland, see your doctor. Proper diagnosis is vital to effective treatment.

Psoriasis

Description And Causes

Skin cells turn over about every 30 days. This means that new skin cells from the lowest layer of the skin are pushed up to the top to replace the dead cells on the surface. With psoriasis, this process happens too quickly, in a matter of days versus a full month. Psoriasis is a type of autoimmune condition where immune cells attack healthy skin cells by mistake. The immune system thinks it is healing a wound or fighting an infection. Because of the rapid turnover, dead skin cells can't slough off quick enough so they build up and form thick, scaly patches on the skin's surface.

The degree of psoriasis symptoms can vary dramatically from one person to the next. In some cases, it is merely a nuisance, while in others it can significantly affect the quality of life. Symptoms of psoriasis can include:

- red patches covered with silvery scales
- dry, cracked skin that can sometimes bleed
- itching, burning, and pain
- swollen and stiff joints
- thick, pitted, or ridged fingernails

Psoriasis can flare during times of stress, while taking certain medications, or if there is an infection present. Dry skin will also worsen psoriasis. Family history can sometimes cause a genetic predisposition to psoriasis.

Treatment

Primary treatments of psoriasis include topical creams, prescription medications, and light therapy. According to MayoClinic.com, treatment can be challenging because "the disease is unpredictable, going through cycles of improvement and worsening seemingly at whim." Weight gain can cause psoriasis to flare. Alcohol, sugar, caffeine, white flour, and wheat can also worsen symptoms in some cases.

The goals of treatment are to stop the rapid turnover of the skin cells and remove scales. All-natural skin creams and light therapy should be considered as first line treatment choices because they are the least toxic. Some drugs used to treat psoriasis, such as methotrexate or azathioprine, have side effects including potential liver damage, nausea, vomiting, and fatigue.

There are many natural substances that can help alleviate the symptoms of psoriasis. Probiotic topical creams can help control the condition. Essential Formulas Incorporated distributes a special line of probiotic skin care products developed by Dr. Ohhira. Other effective ingredients in topical creams include aloe vera, capsaicin (from cayenne), and tea tree oil. Fish oil supplements and evening primrose oil capsules have been shown to be effective in some cases. Curcumin to ease inflammation and silymarin to support effective liver detoxification are also recommended.

An entire treatment protocol for this and many other common skin conditions can be found in Dr. Pescatore's book *The Allergy and Asthma Cure.*

Peptic Ulcer (*see* Ulcers)

Traveler's Diarrhea

Description And Causes

Each year about 10 million people are stricken with traveler's diarrhea. According to the Centers for Disease Control and Prevention (CDC), it is the most common illness effecting travelers. It typically happens within the first week of travel, but it can occur even after returning home. High-risk destinations for traveler's diarrhea include Africa, Asia, Latin America, and the Middle East. The primary cause is the ingestion of fecally- contaminated food or water. The CDC says individuals at high-risk of developing traveler's diarrhea include:

- immunosuppressed individuals
- people with inflammatory bowel disease
- diabetics
- individuals taking H2 blockers or antacids
- young adults

Someone with traveler's diarrhea experiences four to five loose stools a day. It usually begins abruptly and can also cause nausea, vomiting, abdominal cramping, bloating, and fever.

Treatment

Most cases of traveler's diarrhea resolve within one to two days without treatment. Approximately 90 percent of all cases resolve within a week and 98 percent within one month. Staying hydrated is very important. Antibiotics can be given in some cases of severe traveler's diarrhea that is accompanied by severe cramping, fever, and blood in the stool.

Probiotics can help prevent traveler's diarrhea. In an analysis of 12 different clinical trials involving probiotics and the prevention of traveler's diarrhea, researcher Lynne McFarland, PhD, with the VA Puget Sound Health Care System in Seattle, Washington, found that probiotics were very effective in preventing traveler's diarrhea. When traveling, we suggest you pack Dr. Ohhira's brand of probiotics because it is both effective and does not need to be refrigerated.

Ulcers

Description And Causes

Ulcers are sores in the lining of the digestive tract. The most common places for these sores to develop are in the stomach or the duodenum (first part of the intestines). There are three main causes of ulcers:

- *H. pylori* bacteria
- Excess acid and other stomach juices
- NSAID use (aspirin and ibuprofen)

Smoking, alcohol, stress, and diet can make the symptoms of ulcers much worse. Burning pain is the most common symptom. The pain can come and go. It can be worse on an empty stomach and then may go away after eating. With a duodenal ulcer you will feel better when you eat, but worse one to two hours later. With a stomach ulcer you will feel worse when you eat. Other signs of an ulcer include:

- feel full fast
- stomach pain that wakes you up at night
- bloating, burning, or a dull pain in your stomach
- unexpected weight loss
- vomiting

Your ulcer may be getting worse if your pain radiates to your back, you have blood in your vomit or stool, or you frequently feel cold and clammy. For a definitive diagnosis, your doctor may do an endoscopy, which involves a camera that is inserted down your throat and into your stomach.

Treatment

Antibiotics may be prescribed. Other medicines include H2 blockers and proton pump inhibitors. These medicines are designed to reduce the amount of acid your stomach produces. Antacids also neutralize stomach acid. These drugs are not without their side effects, so weigh your options carefully.

An effective natural alternative to conventional ulcer medicines is an extract of licorice known as DGL. Glycyrrhetinic acid in licorice can raise blood pressure, however, deglycyrrhizinated licorice (DGL) removes this toxic compound. The most significant aspect of DGL is that it must be chewed in order to be effective. Although there have not been new clinical studies on this product for several decades, the previous studies were strong and there are lots of testimonial evidence that shows DGL can help many people heal their ulcers.

If you have an ulcer you should avoid spicy foods, avoid dairy (because it is a known food allergen in many people), try not to use aspirin, don't smoke or drink alcohol, reduce the amount of spicy foods in your diet, eat smaller meals, temporarily reduce the number of nutritional supplements you take, and practice stress reduction techniques.

Ulcerative Colitis (*see* Colitis)

Vaginitis

Description And Causes

When the vagina becomes inflamed, it is known as vaginitis. This inflammation is typically caused by a bacterial or yeast infection. Symptoms of vaginitis include:

- change in the color, odor or amount of discharge from the vagina
- vaginal itching and burning
- pain during intercourse
- painful urination
- light vaginal bleeding

The discharge can be different depending on what is causing the vaginitis. With a bacteria infection, the discharge is grayish-white and the odor is stronger. With a yeast infection, the discharge is thick and white. With trichomoniasis (a common sexually-transmitted disease), it is greenish yellow and sometimes frothy.

Bacterial vaginitis is caused by an imbalance of bad to good bacteria in the vagina. A yeast infection is caused by the *C. albicans* fungus and is also known as candidiasis.

Antibiotic use can cause vaginitis. It can also be caused by allergic reactions to spermicides, vaginal hygiene products, detergents, and fabric softeners. Proper diagnosis is critical. If you feel you may have vaginitis, see your doctor for the correct diagnosis.

Treatment

Innovative research from Gregor Reid and his colleagues at the University of Western Ontario in Canada has clearly shown that probitoics can help maintain and restore normal bacterial balance in the vagina. The strain Reid has focused on is *lactobaccilus rhamnosus* GG. Other studies have demonstrated that probiotics can benefit women with vaginitis. In addition to probiotics, goldenseal and uva ursi are herbs that have been used to treat vaginal infections.

Conventionally, antifungal drugs, creams, or suppositories are used. It is important to be sure you get the proper diagnosis. Many of these treatments are available over-the-counter, but if you are treating the wrong cause of vaginitis it could delay recovery or lead to complications.

Bacterial Bedrock

The treatment plan for all of these conditions has one common component: Restore proper bacterial balance. As you can see from such a diverse list of conditions, probiotics don't just benefit the digestive system, they benefit the whole body from head to toe. Bacterial balance is the bedrock of a successful treatment plan for most major illness. The way we achieve this is with effective probiotics. As mentioned previously, we recommend Dr. Ohhira's Probiotics 12 PLUS. This probiotic becomes an essential foundation formula when easing symptoms and healing the underlying cause of most major illnesses. Dr. Ohhira's Probiotics 12 PLUS is exclusively distributed in the United States by Essential Formulas Incorporated (www.essentialformulas.com).

In addition to a high quality probiotic, there are other steps you can take to proactively heal from these conditions. The next chapter outlines our comprehensive plan to prevent illness. In many cases, these recommendations are an effective complement to disease treatment as well.

PART FOUR
BACTERIAL BALANCE

11

PREVENTION PLUS

THE HUMAN BODY IS COMPLEX. Many factors influence our health and our ability to prevent illness. Some aspects of disease and disease prevention remain a mystery. For example, why does one person who smoked cigarettes for decades never develop lung cancer while someone who has never smoked dies of the illness? How can a world-class athlete die of a heart attack when someone who is obese and sedentary never develops a heart condition? When it comes to our health, there are no guarantees.

When we try to prevent illness, we look at improving our odds. We look at ratios and probability. Ultimately, the goal is not about preventing death, it is about enhancing life. Our disease prevention plan will do just that.

Six steps to good health

As we have described, bacteria play a significant role in whether or not we will be sick or well. After all, the human body is made up of far more bacteria than cells. It's not surprising then that bacteria influence a wide range of illnesses that go way beyond the digestive tract.

Having more bad than good bacteria may make our bones thinner, our bodies fatter, and our minds sadder. Bacterial imbalance may negatively influence our metabolism, hormones, brain function, inflammatory response, insulin levels, and immunity. We are just beginning to uncover the far-reaching effects of bacteria and their influence on illness.

Because of this, bacteria are a focal point of our health promotion plan. We not only include good bacteria in our plan, we make sure to support healthy bacterial balance with a comprehensive diet, lifestyle changes, and dietary supplementation. The question that motivated the creation of this plan was: What can we do to support the health and viability of our billion best friends? When we support healthy bacterial balance, we not only prevent illness, we achieve optimum wellness and a higher quality of life. And it all begins with diet.

STEP ONE: Food For Thought

Food is powerful. It has significant influence on our health and even our actions. Have you ever gotten tired in the afternoon after consuming a large, high-carbohydrate lunch? How do you feel after that sugar or caffeine buzz begins to wear off? What happens if you eat too much pepperoni pizza? Our bodies are quick to tell us we've eaten unhealthy foods. The flip side is also true. We get different signals when we eat healthy food. We have more energy, we can think more clearly, we sleep more soundly, and our mood seems to improve.

The reaction to the foods we eat is actually feedback from bacteria in our bodies. If we eat poorly, our good bacteria feel the consequences and try to tell us to stop. And when we eat healthfully, the good bacteria reward us.

Just like us, bacteria need to eat to stay alive and thrive. Good bacteria prefer to eat prebiotics—food that provides them with nourishment. Prebiotics, alone or in conjunction with probiotics, have been clinically studied to provide a whole host of health

Skip The Fries

Sadly, French fries are a vegetable. But once that potato hits the deep fryer, any semblance of nutritive value vanishes. In fact, French fries are one of the most toxic foods you can eat. In addition to being high in trans or saturated fat, French fries contain acrylamides, a cancer-causing substance that is created when starchy foods are cooked at high temperatures. Acrylamides damage cellular DNA. However, the polyphenols found in tea and resveratrol from red grapes have been shown to inhibit acrylamide-induced damage. To avoid acrylamides, always remember to fry foods using healthy oils such as MacNut oil.

benefits that include both the prevention and treatment of serious illnesses. Prebiotic carbohydrates occur naturally in a variety of healthy foods including:

- berries
- garlic
- onions
- flaxseed
- leeks
- dandelion greens
- spinach
- kale
- tomatoes
- lentils
- chickpeas
- black beans

We are often told to eat more of these foods because they are high in fiber and contain important antioxidants. These foods also contain important vitamins and minerals. Perhaps their most significant health benefit, however, is that they provide nourishment to probiotics so those good bacteria can thrive and survive in the body.

Notice there are a variety of greens listed. Eating the right green foods is critical. Many people feel they are eating healthfully when they have a salad with iceberg lettuce. However, iceberg lettuce has very little nutritional value. And most iceberg lettuce is more white than green. Instead, choose mixed greens, spinach, arugula, chard, or bibb lettuce instead of iceberg. If you add tomatoes, chick peas, onions, and some strawberries, you have the perfect probiotic-promoting salad.

Most people are trying to eat healthy by adding more fruits and vegetables to the diet. But it's the type of fruit and vegetable that is important. For example, instead of having a banana, choose a bowl of berries. The banana has a lot of sugar, but the berries contain valuable flavonoid compounds. Instead of choosing white potatoes, choose sweet potatoes. Instead of drinking orange juice, which is also high in sugar, try tomato juice or just eat the orange.

Color is a good indicator that a fruit or vegetable is a healthy choice—the more colorful, the better. Avoid eating meals that are tan and white. Cook with color because the colors confirm the high nutrient content of the fruit or vegetable. The two exceptions to the color rule are onions and garlic. Although both are white (not including the red onion, of course), they are both packed with antioxidants and health-promoting nutrients.

The best way to nourish good bacteria is by feeding them properly. To be healthy and thrive, good bacteria need healthy foods. Eat a minimum of five servings of vegetables every day. That may sound daunting to some people but a serving is not very large. For example, one serving is one of the following:

- 1 cup of leafy greens
- ½ cup of cooked vegetables
- ½ cup fresh vegetable juice

Harmful bacteria thrive in a harsh environment. Remember, earlier in the book we discussed *H. pylori*, which can withstand the

Adding Probiotic to Everything!

Foods high in probiotic bacteria include yogurt, sauerkraut, tempeh, miso, and kefir. Choose organic brands of these foods. Dietary supplements are also a great way to consistently replenish and restore good bacteria.

Not everyone is a fan of yogurt and sauerkraut, and not everyone is taking a probiotic dietary supplement. As a result, creative food manufacturers are trying to slip the good bugs into just about anything they can think of. In 2009, Unilever teamed up with a Finnish ingredient supplier to create a probiotic spread for bread. In addition, a quality probiotic butter is manufactured in Ireland and available in parts of Western Europe. Speaking of bread, a Belgium company has come up with a way to activate prebiotic substances during the baking process of their bread without adding other fibers. As of early 2009, this prebiotic bran bread was not yet on the market in Belgium. Plans to add good bacteria to gum, toothpaste, and even deodorant are also in the works.

In the functional food category, probiotics are taking the market by storm. Be cautious, however. Never choose a food just because it contains good bacteria. Be sure it is low in sugar and does not have preservatives, additives, and fake colors and flavors. Regardless of what takes place in this probiotic food frenzy, the best way to add probiotics to the diet is by taking a quality probiotic supplement every day.

Beyond food, probiotics are also being added to other products as well. Probiotics are a key ingredient in some quality skin care products and will soon be a part of dental products.

onslaught of abrasive acids as it burrows into the stomach lining? Poor nutrition creates a harsh environment that bad bacteria can withstand but good bacteria cannot.

Coincidently, the same foods that help bad bacteria take over also weaken the immune system, cause us to gain weight, and put a strain on the heart. Foods containing sugar and trans fat do the most damage. Highly processed foods and smoked meats containing nitrates are also harmful and should be avoided.

It has been said that one should eat to live not live to eat. As a society, we have become obsessed with food—often the wrong types of food. Our health depends on every forkful of food we eat. Choose wisely and your bacterial buddies will reward you.

Dietary bacterial bottom line: Reduce foods that cause bad bacteria to thrive and increase foods that nourish good bacteria.

STEP TWO: Bathe Your Bacteria

Dehydration is dangerous to your health. Most people are symptom free, yet dehydration is still problematic. Just as plants need water to survive, so do the cells in our bodies. Our good bacteria also need proper hydration. You can live weeks without food, but only days without water.

"Water is the most abundant compound in the human body," says researcher and author Susan M. Kleiner, PhD, RD. "There is no system in the body that does not depend on water."

Water is perhaps one of the most overlooked, yet essential, nutrients we can ingest. It assists with the digestion, absorption, transportation, and use of nutrients. Water helps ensure the safe elimination of waste products and toxic substances. It also enhances enzyme activity and helps lubricate our joints. Without enough water, we are at risk of developing numerous diseases including cancer, arthritis, ulcers, migraines, colitis, and high blood pressure. Dehydration is also linked to low back pain, poor circulation, childhood and adolescent obesity, and poor health in the elderly. A baby's body is made up of about 78 percent water, while an elderly person is only about 50 percent.

Clinical dehydration is a serious medical condition that can cause fatigue, headaches, nosebleeds, infrequent urination, irrational behavior, nausea, intestinal cramping, irregular pulse, and low blood pressure. By the time you experience these symptoms, the dehydration is severe and you should seek medical care. Don't wait until you are thirsty to drink water—by that point you are already dehydrated. Our thirst mechanism turns off when we are chronically dehydrated and our ability to determine our water needs declines with age. Therefore, make drinking water a habit by adding it to your daily routine.

Every day we lose water through sweat, urine, feces, tears, and nasal discharges. We even lose water when we exhale. Some liquids such as coffee, soft drinks, and alcohol are also dehydrating. It has been estimated that we lose about 12 cups of water, even on a cool day without exercising.

Surveys indicate that only about one-third of Americans drink three or fewer servings of water every day. To calculate your water needs, take the number of pounds you weigh and divide that number in half. That number is the fluid ounces you should drink each day. A 200-pound person should drink 100 ounces of water, which is at least twelve 8-ounce cups.

It's critical to drink pure, fresh water. Most municipal tap water should be properly filtered, and even then it may not be completely pure. Municipal water has been shown to contain numerous toxins including harmful bacteria, parasites, lead, arsenic, and prescription drugs. Research the source of your drinking water and be sure it comes from an area that is not tainted by surrounding toxins.

Hydration bacterial bottom line: *Drink a minimum of eight to ten 8-ounce glasses of pure water every day.*

Got Stress?

In today's fast-paced society, it can be hard to relax. Because too much stress or our inability to cope with stress can cause serious health problems, it's worth exploring various relaxation techniques. Here are just a few to choose from.

- **Exercise.** Consistent physical activity is a great way to deal with stress. In addition, exercise helps on so many other levels. Clinical studies show that exercise can help release endorphins, which are positive "feel-good" hormones.

- **Meditation.** This can require lots of practice and maybe even some specific training or classes. Meditation is the act of turning your attention inward to enter a deep state of relaxation. The idea is to clear your head of any thoughts so you can achieve a higher state of self-awareness and relaxation.

- **Visualization.** By visualizing a calm or relaxing place or event, you can achieve a level of peace associated with letting go of the stressful events of the day. The key is to focus on the details and feelings of your relaxing place or event.

- **Progressive muscle relaxation.** This is used to help relieve tense muscles. This technique involves tensing and then relaxing one muscle group at a time. You can do this seated or lying down. Most people start with their lower extremities and then work their way up.

- **Massage.** Seeing a trained massage therapist during times of stress, or on a regular basis, can help alleviate muscle knots. Massage also improves circulation, assists with detoxification, promotes nutrient delivery to tissues, and enhances relaxation.

- **Breathe deeply.** Sometimes when we are under stress we actually forget to breathe or our breathing becomes shallow. Deep breathing from the belly will help relieve stress and deliver more oxygen to the brain. A great deep breathing exercise is to breathe in deeply through your nose for a count of four and then breathe out through your mouth for a count of four. Do this several times a day.

- **Create balance.** The best ways to cope with stress are to learn to say no and schedule time for yourself each day. This will help create balance so you can avoid that "stressed out" feeling.

- **Be positive.** During times of stress, it can be difficult to be upbeat. Try to look for positives in your day. Reframe the way you look at problems and give yourself and others positive messages. Developing a positive attitude can go a long way in coping with stress.

- **Diet and dietary supplements.** Eating healthfully and taking dietary supplements to fill in the gaps will help our bodies cope with added stress. Research featured in the journal Nutrition Research from 2008 demonstrated that taking a probiotic supplement helped reduce stress-induced gastrointestinal symptoms including abdominal pain, nausea, and vomiting.

It's nearly impossible to completely alleviate stress. After all, some positive experiences are stressful like the birth of a child, a new job, or an important celebration. During stressful times there can be a tendency to turn to unhealthy coping methods such as drinking too much alcohol, eating too much, smoking, or not exercising. The key to relaxation is to find health-promoting ways to cope with stress. Surround yourself with loving people and participate in activities that you enjoy such as reading, being in nature, hanging out with friends or a four-legged companion, or journaling. By doing this, you will be offsetting the negative effects that stress can have on your health.

STEP THREE: Actions Speak Loudly

What we do is often more compelling than what we say, especially when it comes to our health. Our actions send clear messages to our bacteria. Health-promoting actions such as exercise and stress reduction strengthen good bacteria, while unhealthy activities such as smoking and eating poorly support harmful bacteria. Being physically active is one of the most significant health-promoting actions you can do for your body.

Exercise not only strengthens muscles and keeps us from getting winded as we climb stairs, it also has many other health benefits that you may not even be aware of. Being physically active will help:

- strengthen your immune system
- improve circulation
- enhance mood and self-image
- increase energy
- improve digestion
- boost brain function
- prevent obesity

That's a pretty impressive list of benefits! When we think of exercise we need to look beyond the spandex stereotypes and muscle-bound weight lifters. Being physically active is just that—being active. There are two aspects that will ensure you get the benefits of exercise:

·**Frequency.** It is better to be physically active four days a week for 30 minutes rather than twice a week for an hour.

Have fun. Choose physical activities that you enjoy and don't be afraid to mix it up to keep it interesting.

Take the stairs, go for a walk at lunchtime, dig in your garden on the weekends, or take your dog or your kids to the park after work. Whatever it takes, add activity to your day.

Scientific research has proven beyond a doubt that being physically active will help prevent a wide range of health ailments including arthritis, diabetes, Alzheimer's, heart disease, and cancer. One of the most significant "side effects" of exercise is weight loss. Taking a 50-minute walk will burn about 250 calories. In addition, exercise provides powerful stress relief. This is significant because stress has been linked to a weakened immune system, disturbed digestive tract, and dangerous heart conditions. For more information on stress reduction, refer to the side bar on pages 200-201.

To get the most out of your physical fitness program, include activities in these three areas:

- cardiovascular, which involves the heart and the lungs
- muscular strength and endurance
- flexibility

In addition to popular exercise classes such as step aerobics or weight training, you can try Pilates, yoga, or Tai Chi. You can swim, ski, hike, bike, or horseback ride. When you think of exercise merely as movement, it makes it more universally accessible.

If you have been inactive for a long period of time, check with your doctor before embarking on a new exercise program and begin slowly. If you are already an active person, try increasing the intensity, duration, and frequency of your activity. To avoid plateaus and potential frustration, add new activities and rotate them.

Although exercise will help ease insomnia, you should avoid exercising late in the evening because it could have the opposite effect. Gentle stretching or yoga in the evening is a better choice because it will help you unwind, relax, and sleep soundly.

Susan Ryan, DO, is board certified in both sports medicine and family practice. She sums up the value of exercise this way: "Exercise not only adds years to your life, it also adds life to your years."

Lifestyle bacterial bottom line: Be as physically active as possible.

STEP FOUR: Sleep Soundly

Don't underestimate the significant value of a good night's sleep. When you think of sleep, you may think it is a time of inactivity—when our bodies can wind down from the day's events. But that's not the case. When we sleep soundly, there is a whirlwind of activity inside our bodies as we repair muscles, release hormones, bolster immunity, and energize our cells. Sleep affects our ability to concentrate, our moods, and even how we look. In fact, new research shows that lack of sleep can make you fat.

According to the *International Journal of Obesity*, individuals who are sleep-deprived have more body fat than those who sleep well. "These associations persisted after adjusting for sleep apnea, insomnia, and daytime sleepiness," concluded the researchers. In other words, even if you don't have a diagnosed sleep disorder, you can still experience the damaging affects of sleep deprivation. The researchers also found that shortened sleep cycles were associated with a higher body fat percentage, as well as a wider waistline.

While we sleep, chemicals and hormones that help control appetite are released. If we are not sleeping soundly, those chemical messengers and hormones are disrupted, which can cause us to gain weight.

Eve Van Cauter, PhD, professor of medicine at the University of Chicago says "chronic sleep loss may not only hasten the onset, but could also increase the severity, of age-related ailments such as diabetes, hypertension, obesity, and memory loss."

In addition, lack of sleep is associated with depression, anxiety, and even accelerated aging. The most common sleep complaint is insomnia affecting about one-third of the American population, with women more than twice as likely to experience it than men.

Many people are not getting the recommended seven to nine hours of sound sleep per night. Do all of those people have insomnia? If you have difficulty falling asleep, can't stay asleep, or are

The Myth of Pulling an "All-Nighter"

Remember when we were in school and we were cramming for an important exam? Many of us would "pull an all-nighter," forgoing our need for sleep as we overstuffed our brains with valuable information. Deep down, we knew what the researchers are now confirming—exhaustion leads to memory loss and a poor grade on the exam. Even today, some of us stay up all night to meet a work deadline only to find ourselves not sharp enough to deliver the presentation or experiencing fuzzy thinking in our important meeting.

According to Matthew Walker, director of the Sleep and Neuroimaging Lab at the University of California, Berkeley, "Sleep, we've been finding, actually can enhance your memory so you can come back the next day even better than you were the day before."

Sleep is not merely for resting. It serves a broad range of vital purposes. From an evolutionary standpoint, sleep is when both animals and humans are at their most vulnerable. Walker says, if the point is survival, sleep must "be so important that evolution is willing to put us in that place of potential danger. It would be the biggest evolutionary mistake if sleep does not serve some critical function."

experiencing poor sleep quality three nights a week for more than a month, you have insomnia.

Some people have what's known as stress-induced insomnia, when the stress of everyday living gets in the way of a good night's sleep. This type of insomnia can be difficult to manage because we often can't simply remove the stressor, such as money problems or job pressures.

Insomnia can be maddening. As a result, many people turn to over-the-counter (OTC) and prescription drugs. These drugs are not without side effects, which can include dependence, confusion, dry mouth, and morning drowsiness. Some individuals can experience allergic reactions and these drugs can interact negatively with pain-killers, sedatives, other drugs, and alcohol. Withdrawal from sleeping medications can also cause nausea and a worsening of insomnia. Never discontinue taking prescription medications without first consulting with your doctor. Fortunately, there are many natural ingredients that can provide a viable—and safe—alternative to OTC and prescription sleeping pills.

For those suffering from chronic insomnia, just drinking a cup of chamomile tea in the evening is often not enough. Melatonin is best known as a natural cure for jet lag, however, many studies have shown it to be very effective for insomnia. A 2008 study demonstrated that 5 mg of melatonin daily helped shift working nurses fall asleep faster. The newest information regarding melatonin is that a controlled-release form of melatonin is proving to be even more effective. In 2008 a report in the journal *Expert Opinion on Investigational Drugs* showed that a prolonged-released melatonin significantly improved morning alertness and sleep quality in patients over age 55.

Gamma-aminobutyric acid, also known as GABA, is an amino acid proven to be an effective natural insomnia treatment. In 2008, researchers from Brigham & Women's Hospital showed that non-medicated individuals suffering from insomnia have significantly lower levels of GABA in the brain.

In 1990, tryptophan was taken off the market due to contamination. Today, pure, pharmaceutical-grade L-tryptophan is back on the market so people can take advantage of this powerful natural substance. L-tryptophan is an amino acid that has been shown to naturally enhance sleep. L-tryptophan crosses the blood-brain barrier where it is converted to serotonin and later further metabolized into melatonin.

For stress-induced insomnia, try L-theanine. "For several years, I have been impressed that Suntheanine [a brand of L-theanine] is the only substance, natural or otherwise, that reduces feelings of stress and improves sleep quality without creating drowsiness or diminished motor performance," explains Michael R. Lyon, MD, Medical and Research Director of the Canadian Center for Functional Medicine with the University of British Columbia.

In addition to achieving seven to nine hours of sleep each night, it is important to experience quality sleep with fewer nighttime awakenings and less restlessness. For this, you can try 3 mg daily of vitamin B12 (methylcobalamin). Studies show that methylcobalamin improves sleep quality, increases feelings of alertness during the day, and helps individuals feel refreshed upon waking in the morning.

In addition to dietary supplements, people who have difficulty sleeping may want to try the following dietary and lifestyle tips to help ensure consistent, sound slumber:

- Establish a regular bedtime and wake time.
- Reserve the bedroom for intimacy and sleep only. Do not watch television, eat, talk on the phone, or work in your bedroom.
- Make your bedroom dark, quiet, and comfortable.
- Avoid caffeine and alcohol before bedtime; drink calming teas instead.
- Avoid sugary foods and refined carbohydrates before bedtime.
- Avoid foods with additives and preservatives because some of these ingredients can act as stimulants.
- To avoid nighttime awakening due to drops in blood sugar, eat a small amount of nuts or celery with cheese before retiring so the blood sugar effect lasts well into the night.

We spend about one-third of our lives sleeping. That's because the body needs that time to replenish, restore, and rejuvenate on the cellular level. It only makes sense to maximize that time. Dietary supplements can help enhance the quantity and quality of our sleep. This will ensure that our bodies are ready to tackle another day. If you sleep well, you will be well.

Sleep bacterial bottom line: *Don't underestimate the health-promoting effects of getting seven to nine hours of sleep each night.*

STEP FIVE: Supplemental Insurance

Dietary supplements are just that, supplements to the diet. But that doesn't mean we can eat horribly, then simply pop a pill to offset the damage. Supplements should not take the place of healthy foods. They are designed to complement the diet. We need the nutrients provided by dietary supplements to enhance our diet and fill in the gaps. Every individual, even those who pay very close attention to what they eat, may need to take dietary supplements. Depleted soil and food processing negatively impacts the nutrient content of our food. In addition, high stress levels, lack of sleep, and other factors can increase our demands for dietary supplements.

Certain individuals may require more dietary supplementation than others including:
- individuals struggling with a specific illness
- the elderly
- women who are pregnant or nursing
- children
- people who are under a lot of stress
- those with a family history of serious illness

If you fall into one or more of these categories, you may want to consider getting some advice from a holistic-minded physician or naturopathic doctor. However, whether you have special nutritional needs or not, we feel every individual will benefit from taking three key dietary supplements. These three supplements provide a strong nutritional foundation to build upon and will help enhance a healthy diet and lifestyle. They include:

- A high-quality multi-vitamin/mineral supplement.
- A fish oil supplement that contains essential fatty acids, specifically DHA and EPA (vegans can us a plant oil essential fatty acid in place of fish oils).
- A probiotic that contains bacterial strains that have been scientifically proven to be effective, as well as prebiotic ingredients (as mentioned previously).

Because of the various bacterial issues we have described in this book, probiotics should be used just as you would a multi-vitamin/mineral supplement—taken daily. The body does manufacture these good bacteria, however, since they are constantly being attacked by our unhealthy lifestyle, we must get them from food and dietary supplements. We must also replenish them on a daily basis if we are to get the full health-promoting, disease-preventing benefits they provide.

Depending on your individual circumstances, you can add other dietary supplements as appropriate. For example, if you have peptic ulcers, you may want to try chewable DGL. Or if you are under a great deal of stress, you may choose L-theanine. If you are taking a prescription medication, never discontinue taking that medication without first talking with your doctor. You should also always tell your doctor what dietary supplements you are taking. For example, garlic and ginkgo may act as blood thinners and should not be taken before surgery because they could cause excessive bleeding. The three dietary supplements we recommend are safe to use with other supplements and OTC or prescription medications.

Dietary supplements should be taken in divided dosages rather than a high dose just once a day. When purchasing a dietary supplement, don't skimp. This is not the time to choose the cheapest, it's the time to choose the best. Pick brands that you can trust.

Dietary supplements are not drugs, so it may take a little while before you see results; however, if you are not feeling better after taking a dietary supplement for a few weeks, you may want to consider another brand. When used in conjunction with a healthy diet and lifestyle, dietary supplements can make a world of difference.

Some people may experience a "healing crisis" when taking some supplements. This means you may actually feel worse before you feel better. Don't panic, this is common in certain circumstances.

Increased toxins, stress, fast food, food processing, and many other factors have created a critical need for dietary supplements. When used prudently, dietary supplements can help you prevent illness.

Dietary supplement bacterial bottom line: Take a high-quality probiotic supplement, multi-vitamin mineral formula, and essential fatty acids.

STEP SIX: Believe in Balance

This entire book has been about balance—the balance of good versus bad bacteria, and tipping the scales in favor of the good. Let's apply that same philosophy to our proactive prevention plan.

From a percentage standpoint, the goal is to have 80 to 85 percent good bacteria and 15 to 20 percent bad. If you follow the guidelines provided in this book at least 80 percent of the time, you are dramatically improving your chances of being healthy. It's about balance.

You now understand that you have access to billions of bacteria that can work on your behalf to be healthy. If you support them properly, they will do their job. They will be the best friends you will ever have. Bacterial balance is the missing link to disease prevention and living life with vitality.

Bacterial balance bottom line: *Support healthy bacterial balance in everything you do.*

The Future of Healthcare

The last time your doctor prescribed an antibiotic, did he/she also recommend a probiotic supplement? Chances are the answer is no. Our healthcare system is not set up to encourage doctors to dispense, or even recommend, dietary supplements. For decades, doctors have received very little training on diet and the health implications associated with the foods we eat. That's changed somewhat.

Our healthcare system is broken and nobody is likely to argue that fact. Until things change with healthcare delivery, pharmaceutical influence, and medical education, patients and doctors are left to take the lead. Patients must become more responsible and proactive, and doctors must become more open-minded. The proper shift can help each meet in the middle, speaking the same language—a language of integration and collaboration.

When our healthcare system is fixed, we will no longer see division and an "either-or" mentality. The pharmacist will ask the patient if they are taking a quality probiotic as he/she hands the antibiotic prescription to the patient. The patient will feel safe to tell the doctor about the dietary supplements they are taking. There will not be descriptive labels such as "conventional medicine" or "complementary or alternative", there will just be good medicine.

Understanding and embracing the expansive influence of both good and bad bacteria is just the beginning. It is a step towards the middle, where things are not black and white. It is a step towards a future healthcare system that values prevention as much as treatment.

Let's Review

To support your billion best friends, focus on the following:

- A diet that features lots of fresh, green leafy vegetables and low sugar fruits.

- Drinking plenty of fresh, pure water every day.

- Consistent physical activity.

- Rest, relaxation, and sound sleep.

- Dietary supplements, specifically a multi-vitamin/mineral formula, essential fatty acids, and a probiotic.

- Balance all of the above with a healthy dose of occasional indulgence.

TERMS TO KNOW

Antibiotic: A substance that inhibits the growth of or destroys bacterial microorganisms.

Antibiotic Resistance: The ability of microorganism to not be destroyed by an antibiotic.

Bacteria: Any living single-cell microorganism, some of which can cause disease.

Bacterial Species: Classification of bacteria that further describes them beyond their genus.

Bacterial Strain: A subset of a bacterial species.

Colony Forming Units (CFUs): A measure of viable bacterial cells in a colony representing an aggregate of those cells derived from a single originating bacteria.

Culture: The process by which bacterial cells are grown under controlled conditions.

Digestion: The process that transports ingested food through the digestive system to process and break it down into nutrients that can be absorbed, or turn it into waste material that can be eliminated.

Digestive System: The organs and systems involved with ingestion, digestion, absorption, and defecation.

Dysbiosis: Bacterial imbalance characterized by an overgrowth of harmful bacteria.

Fermentation: The process by which cells release energy, bringing about a chemical change.

Flora: Bacteria living in or on the body.

Fungi: Neither plant nor animal, fungi such as mushrooms or molds are micro-organisms that belong to the fungal kingdom.

Gastroenterology: The branch of medicine that studies the digestive system and disorders of the gastrointestinal tract, which include the organs from the mouth to the anus.

Gut: This is another term for the digestive tract, which is the hollow tube that stretches from the mouth to the anus.

Human Microbiome Project: NIH sponsored project to study micro-organisms present in or on five different parts of the human body using living volunteers.

Lactic acid bacteria: Used to ferment food, lactic acid bacteria produce lactic acid.

Leaky Gut Syndrome: Thinning of the intestinal wall, allowing toxins and large particles to enter the blood stream.

Microbe: A microscopic organism that transmits disease.

Microbiome: The group of associated microflora in a human.

Microflora: Microscopic living bacterial colonies found in the intestines.

Microorganism: A minute living organism, such as bacteria or viruses, that can only be seen under a microscope.

Oligosaccharides: Any group of carbohydrates consisting of a small number of simple sugar molecules; most commercial prebiotics are oligosaccharides.

Parasite: An organism that lives in or on a host and obtains nourishment from the host.

Prebiotic: Functional food items that stimulate the growth of good bacteria.

Probiotic: Beneficial bacteria similar to the friendly bacteria in the intestines.

Species: See bacterial species.

Strain: See bacterial strain.

Synbiotic: A dietary supplement that contains one or more prebiotics and probiotics that work synergistically.

Vegan: Someone who does not eat animal, dairy products, or fish.

Vegetarian: Someone who does not consume animal products; there are many subsets depending on the person.

Virus: A microscopic infectious agent that is unable to live outside of a host; viruses cannot be killed by antibiotics.

Yeast: A single cell fungi used to leaven bread, and also found in cheese and other fermented foods and beverages.

Selected references
by chapter

Chapter 1

http://www.ucmp.berkeley.edu/history/leeuwenhoek.html

http://astrobio.net/news/article2447.html

http://archives.cnn.com/2000/HEALTH/06/01/antibiotic.overuse/index.html

http://enews.tufts.edu/stories/102/2007/10/29/MakingSenseofMRSA

http://www.emedicinehealth.com/antibiotics/page4_em.htm

http://www.microbeworld.org/microbes/bacteria

http://www.cdc.gov/cogh/dgphcd/modules/ddm/ch1_ch.htm

http://www.cdc.gov/h1n1flu/swineflue_you.htm

http://www.functionalingredientsmag.com

Adler, Jerry and Jeneen Interlandi. Caution: Killing germs may be hazardous to your health. *Newsweek*. Oct 29, 2007.

Donn, Jeff, et al. AP Probe Finds Drugs in Drinking Water. *Associated Press*. March 10, 2008.

Grice EA, et al. A diversity profile of the human skin microbiota. *Genome Research*. 18(7):1043-50, 2008.

Gross PA, Patel B. Reducing antibiotic overuse: a call for a national performance measure for not treating asymptomatic bacteriuria. *Clinical Infectious Disease*. 45(10):1335-7, 2007.

Johnson S, et al. Epidemics of diarrhea caused by a clindamycin-resistant strain of clostridium difficile in four hospitals. *The New England Journal of Medicine*. 22(341):1645-1651, 1999.

Ladd E. The use of antibiotics for viral upper respiratory tract infections: an analysis of nurse practitioner and physician prescribing practices in ambulatory care, 1997-2001. *Journal of the American Academy of Nurse Practitioners.* 17(10):416-24, 2005.

Margolis DJ, et al. Effects of antibiotics on the oropharyngeal flora in patients with acne. *Archives of Dermatology.* 139(4):467-471, 2003.

Margolis DJ, et al. Antibiotic treatment of acne may be associated with upper respiratory tract infections. *Archives of Dermatology.* 141(9):1131-1136, 2005.

Murray, Michael T. *Natural Alternatives to Over-the-Counter and Prescription Drugs.* New York: William Morrow, 1994.

Ryan, Susan. Emergency room physician at Rose Medical Center in Denver, CO. Telephone interview on March 5, 2008.

Sachs, Jessica Snyder. *Good Germs, Bad Germs: Health and survival in a bacterial world.* New York: Hill and Wang, 2007.

Steinman MA, et al. Predictors of broad-spectrum antibiotic prescribing for acute respiratory tract infections in adult primary care. *Journal of the American Medical Association.* 289(6):719-25, 2003.

Torkos, Sherry. Integrative pharmacist in Canada. E-mail correspondence April 2, 2008.

Velicer CM, et al. Antibiotic use in relation to the risk of breast cancer. *Journal of the American Medical Association.* 291(7):827-35, 2004.

Zugler, Abigail. Separating friend from foe among the body's invaders. *The New York Times.* Nov 27, 2007.

Chapter 2

http://genome.wustl.edu/sub_genome_group.cgi?GROUP = 3&SUB_GROUP = 4

http://www.microbeworld.org

http://64.233.169.104/search?q = cache:kBsuXRpmNi0J:digestive.niddk.nih.gov/about/ddnews/win08/DD_Newsltr-winter08.pdf + James + Gordon, + MD, + bacteria + and + weight + loss&hl = en&ct = clnk&cd = 6&gl = us&client = safari

Collins FS, National Human Genome Research Institute Director and a co-chair of the Human Microbiome Project Implementation Group, personal e-mail correspondence. June 2008.

Grice EA, et al. A diversity profile of the human skin microbiota. *Genome Research.* 18(7):1043-50, 2008.

Hayes CS, Williamson H. Management of Group A Beta-Hemolytic Streptococcal Pharyngitis. *American Family Physician.* 63:1557-64, 2001.

Hoffman RL. Probiotics: Twenty-first century support for healthy digestive and immune systems. *Townsend Letter.* Feb/Mar 2007.

Hooton TM, Levy SB. Antimicrobial Resistance: A plan of action for community practice. *American Family Physician*. 63:1087-96, 2001.

Krensky, Alán M. Telephone interview on Aug 27, 2008.

Sachs, Jessica Snyder. *Good Germs, Bad Germs: Health and survival in a bacterial world*. New York: Hill and Wang 2007.

Chapter 3

http://www.bt.cdc.gov/disasters/handhygienefacts.asp

http://www.cdc.gov/salmonella/

http://www.organicconsumers.org/foodsafety/shortlist031604.cfm

http://www.ucsusa.org/food_and_environment/antibiotics_and_food/european-union-ban.html

http://www.ota.com/organic/foodsafety/OrganicBeef.html

http://www.ota.com/organic/mt/business.html

http://digestive.niddk.nih.gov/ddiseases/topics/diagnostic.asp

http://enews.tufts.edu/stories/102/2007/10/29/MakingSenseofMRSA/print

http://www.chicagotribune.com/business/chi-tue-mcdonalds-tomatoes-salmonella-jun09,0,4285616.story

http://www.nytimes.com/2007/12/06/business/06meat.html?ei = 5070&en = 54e0fa8bbcb3fl&oref = slogin

Adler, Jerry and Jeneen Interlandi. Caution: Killing germs may be hazardous to your health. *Newsweek*. Oct 29, 2007.

Gittleman, Ann Louise. *The Gut Flush Plan*. New York: Avery Publishing, 2008.

Hooton TM, Levy SB. Antimicrobial Resistance: A plan of action for community practice. *American Family Physician*. 63:1087-98, 2001.

Klevens RM, et al. Invasive methicillin-resistant Staphylococcus aureus infection in the United States. *Journal of the American Medical Association*. 298(15):1763-71, 2007.

Mehrotra A, et al. Preventive health examinations and preventive gynecological examinations in the United States. *Archives of Internal Medicine*. 167(17):1876-83, Sept 2007.

Sachs, Jessica Snyder. *Good Germs, Bad Germs: Health and survival in a bacterial world*. New York: Hill and Wang 2007.

Sandora TJ, et al. Reducing absenteeism from gastrointestinal and respiratory illness in elementary school students: A randomized, controlled trial of an infection-control intervention. *Pediatrics*. 121(6):1555-1562, 2008.

Chapter 4

http://nccam.nih.gov/health/probiotics/

http://digestive.niddk.nih.gov/about/ddnews/win08/1.htm

http://www.lifeclinic.com/focus/nutrition/food-pyramid.asp

http://www.nutraingredients.com/content/view/print/244976

Bromstein E. Gut reaction to probiotics: Beware some of those touted living organisms could be dead. *NOW Magazine online*. Oct 18-24, 2007.

DiBaise JK, et al. Gut microbiota and its possible relationship with obesity. *Mayo Clinic Proceedings*. 83(4):460-9, 2008.

McFarland LV. Beneficial microbes: health or hazard? *European Journal of Gastroenterology & Hepatology*. 12(10):1069-71, 2000.

Parnell JA, Reimer RA. Weight loss during oligofructose supplementation is associated with decreased ghrelin and increased peptide YY in overweight and obese adults. *Am J Clin Nutr* 89(6):1751-9, June 2009.

Reid, Gregor. E-mail correspondence. February 2008.

Szajewska H, et al. Probiotics in gastrointestinal diseases in children: hard and not-so-hard evidence of efficacy. *Journal of Pediatric Gastroenterology and Nutrition*. 42(5):454-75. 2006.

Turnbaugh PJ, et al. Diet-induced obesity is linked to marked but reversible alterations in the mouse distal gut microbiome. *Cell Host & Microbe*. 3(4):213-23, 2008.

Yoo SS, et al. The human emotional brain without sleep: A prefrontal-amygdala disconnect. *Current Biology*. 17(20): 877-878, 2007.

Chapter 5

Arslanoglu S, et al. Early dietary intervention with a mixture of prebiotic oligosaccharides reduces the incidence of allergic manifestations and infections during the first two years of life. *Journal of Nutrition*. 138(6):1091-5, 2008.

Bouhnik Y, et al. The capacity of short-chain fructo-oligosaccharides to stimulate faecal bifidobacteria: a dose-response relationship study in healthy humans. *Nutrition Journal*. 5(8), 2006.

Duc le H, et al. Characterization of Bacillus probiotics available for human use. *Applied and Environmental Microbiology*. 70(4):2161-71, 2004.

Hoa NT, et al. Characterization of Bacillus species used for oral bacteriotherapy and bacterioprophylaxis of gastrointestinal disorders. *Applied and Environmental Microbiology*. 66(12):5241-7, Dec 2000.

Hong HA, et al. The use of bacterial spore formers as probiotics. *FEMS Microbiology Review*. 29(4):813-35, 2005.

Lin JS, et al. Different effects of probiotic species/strains on infections in preschool children: A double-blind, randomized, controlled study. *Vaccine*. 27(7):1073-9, 2009.

Szajewska H, et al. Probiotics in gastrointestinal diseases in children: hard and not-so-hard evidence of efficacy. *Journal of Pediatric Gastroenterology and Nutrition* 42(5):454-75, 2006.

Chapter 6

http://www.consumerlab.com/results/probiotics.asp

http://www.medicalnewstoday.com/printerfriendlynews.php?newsid = 117664

Friedrich MJ. Benefits of gut microflora under study. *Journal of the American Medical Association*. 299(2), 2008.

Lenoir-Wijnkoop I, et al. Probiotic and prebiotic influence beyond the intestinal tract. *Nutrition Review*. 65(11):469-89, 2007.

Ouwehand AC. Antiallergic effects of probiotics. *Journal of Nutrition*. 137:794S-7S, 2007.

Scholz-Ahrens KE, et al. Prebiotics, probiotics, and synbiotics affect mineral absorption, bone mineral content, and bone structure. *Journal of Nutrition*. 137:838S-46S, 2007.

Sleater RD, Hill C. Probiotics as therapeutics for the developing world. *Journal of Infection in Developing Countries*. 1(1):7-12, 2007.

Sleater RD, Hill C. Patho-biotechnology: Using bad bugs to do good things. *Current Opinion in Biotechnology*. 17(2):211-6, 2006.

Chapter 7

http://www.ornl.gov/sci/techresources/Human_Genome/elsi/gmfood.shtml

http://www.ota.com/organic/benefits/generic.html

Elson CO. From Cheese to Pharma: A designer probiotic for IBD. *Clinical Gastroenterology and Hepatology*. 4(7):836-7, 2006.

Gittleman, Ann Louise. *The Gut Flush Plan*. New York: Avery Publishing, 2008.

Laldoria HT, Gatcheco FN. The effect of probiotics in the treatment of acute non-bloody diarrhea in infants aged 3 to 24 months. *The First Congress of Asian Society for Pediatric Research*, Nov 2005.

Ohhira, Iichiroh. E-mail interview correspondence, June 2008.

Ohhira I, et al. Identification of 3-Phenyllactic Acid As a Possible Antibacterial Substance Produced by Enterococcus faecalis TH10. *Biocontrol Science*. 9(3):77-81, 2004.

Ohhira I. Studies on Lactic Acid Bacteria Enterococcus faecalis TH10, Biobank Co., Ltd., 2003.

Pelton, Ross. E-mail interview correspondence, March 2008.

Quigley, Eamonn. E-mail interview correspondence, March 2008.

Reid, Gregor. E-mail interview correspondence, February 2008.

Sleator RD, Hill C. Bioengineered Bugs—a patho-biotechnology approach to probiotic research and applications. *Medical Hypothesis*. 70(1):167-9, 2007.

Turnbaugh PJ, et al. The Human Microbiome Project. *Nature*. 449(18), 2007.

Chapter 8

http://www.usatoday.com/news/nation/2008-03-10-cities-water_N.htm

www.emaxhealth.com. Altering Bugs in the Gut Could Tackle Non-Alcoholic Fatty Liver Disease, Imperial College of London, August 2006.

Alschuler, Lise, and Karolyn A Gazella. *The Definitive Guide to Cancer*. Berkeley, CA: Celestial Arts, 2007.

Bik EM, et al. Molecular analysis of the bacterial microbiota in the human stomach. *Proceedings of the National Academy of Sciences USA*. 103(7):732-7, 2006.

Bu LN, et al. Lactobacillus casei rhamnosus Lcr35 in children with chronic constipation. *Pediatrics International*. 49(4):485-90, 2007.

Lebrose-Pantoflickova D, et al. Helicobacter pylori and probiotics. *Journal of Nutrition*. 137(3 Suppl):812S-8S, 2007.

Li Z, et al. Probiotics and antibiotics to TNF inhibit inflammatory activitiy and improve nonalcoholic fatty liver disease. *Hepatology*. 37(2):343-50, 2003.

Pradhan SC, Girish C. Hepatoprotective herbal drug, silymarin from experimental pharmacology to clinical medicine. *The Indian Journal of Medical Research*. 124(5):491-504, 2006.

Wellington K, Jarvis B. Silymarin: a review of its clinical properties in the management of hepatic disorders. *BioDrugs*. 15(7):465-89, 2001.

Chapter 9

http://www.wellnessletter.com/html/wl/2008/wlFeatured0608.html

http://www.sciam.com/article.cfm?id = infected-with-insanity

http://www.csaceliacs.org

http://www.nutraingredients.com/content/view/print/243575

Al-Salami H, et al. Probiotic treatment reduces blood glucose levels and increases systemic absorption of gliclazide in diabetic rats. *European Journal of Drug Metabolism and Pharmacokinetics*. 33(2):101-6, 2008.

Cox AJ, et al. Oral administration of the probiotic Lactobacillus fermentum VRI-003 and mucosal immunity in endurance athletes. *British Journal of Sports Medicine.* Published online Feb 2008.

Dogi CA, et al. Gut immune stimulation by non pathogenic Gram(+) and Gram(-) bacteria. Comparison with a probiotic strain. *Cytokine.* 41(3):223-31, Mar 2008.

Forsyth CB, et al. Lactobacillus GG treatment ameliorates alcohol-induced intestinal oxidative stress, gut leakiness, and liver injury in a rat model of alcoholic steatohepatitis. *Alcohol.* 43(2):163-72, 2009.

Guandalini S. Probiotics for children: Use in diarrhea. *Journal of Clinical Gastroenterology.* 40(3):244-8, 2006.

Isolauri E, et al. Probiotics: Effects on immunity. *American Journal of Clinical Nutrition.* 73(2Suppl):444S-450S, 2001.

Ivory K, et al. Oral delivery of Lactobacillus casei Shirota modifies allergen-induced immune responses in allergic rhinitis. *Clinical and Experimental Allergy.* 38(8):1282-9, 2008.

Janiszewski PM, et al. Does waist circumference predict diabetes and cardiovascular disease beyond commonly evaluated cardiometabolic risk factors? *Diabetes Care.* 30(12):3105-9, 2007.

Kirpich IA, et al. Probiotics restore bowel flora and improve liver enzymes in human alcohol-induced liver injury: A pilot study. *Alcohol.* 42(8):675-82, 2008.

Kligler B, et al. Probiotics in children. *Pediatric Clinics of North America.* 54(6):949-67, 2007.

Kodali VP, Sen R. Antioxidant and free radical scavenging activities of an exopolysaccharide from a probiotic bacterium. *Biotechnology Journal.* 3(2):245-51, 2008.

Laitinen K, et al. Probiotics and dietary counseling contribute to glucose regulation during and after pregnancy: A randomized controlled trial. *British Journal of Nutrition.* Published online Nov 2008.

Lin JS, et al. Different effects of probiotic species/strains on infections in preschool children: A double-blind, randomized, controlled study. *Vaccine.* 27(7):1073-9, 2009.

Lowry CA, et al. Identification of an immune-responsive mesolimbocortical serotonergic system: Potential role in regulation of emotional behavior. *Neuroscience.* 146(2):756-72, 2007.

Niers L, et al. The effects of selected probiotic strains on the development of eczema (the PandA study). *Allergy.* Published online April 9, 2009.

Osborn DA, Sinn JK. Probiotics in infants for prevention of allergic disease and food hypersensitivity. *Cochrane Database System Review.* 4:CD006475, Oct 2007.

Ouwehand AC, et al. Influence of a combination of Lactobacillus acidophilus NCFM and lactitol on healthy elderly: Intestinal and immune parameters. *British Journal of Nutrition.* 101(3):367-75, 2009.

Poulain M, et al. The effect of obesity on chronic respiratory diseases: Pathophysiology and therapeutic strategies. *Canadian Medical Association Journal.* 174(9), 2006.

Rao AV, et al. A randomized, double-blind, placebo-controlled pilot study of a probiotic in emotional symptoms of chronic fatigue syndrome. *Gut Pathogens.* 1(1):6, 2009.

Rocha PM, et al. Independent and opposite associations of hip and waist circumference with metabolic syndrome components and with inflammatory and atherothrombotic risk factors in overweight and obese women. *Metabolism.* 57(10):1315-22, 2008.

Saavedra JM, Tschernia A. Human studies with probiotics and prebiotics: Clinical implications. *British Journal of Nutrition.* 87(2Suppl):S241-6, 2002.

Van Baarlen P, et al. Differential NF-kappaB pathways induction by Lactobacillus plantarum in the duodenum of healthy humans correlating with immune tolerance. *Proceedings of the National Academy of Sciences USA.* 106(7):2371-6, 2009.

Wang Y, et al. A prospective study of waist circumference and body mass index in relation to colorectal cancer incidence. *Cancer Causes & Control.*19(7):783-92, 2008.

Wang Y, et al. Comparison of abdominal adiposity and overall obesity in predicting risk of type 2 diabetes among men. *American Journal of Clinical Nutrition.* 81(3):555-63, March 2005.

Yolken RH, Torrey EF. Are some cases of psychosis caused by microbial agents? A review of the evidence. *Molecular Psychiatry.* 13(5):470-9, 2008.

Zhang C, et al. Abdominal obesity and the risk of all-cause, cardiovascular, and cancer mortality: Sixteen years of follow-up in US women. *Circulation.* 117(13):1658-67, 2008.

Chapter 10

http://www.nlm.nih.gov/medlineplus/healthtopics_a.html

http://www.nutraingredients.com/content/view/print/242060

Abrams SA, et al. A combination of prebiotic short- and long-chain inulin-type fructans enhances calcium absorption and bone mineralization in young adolescents. *American Journal of Clinical Nutrition.* 82(2):471-6, 2005.

Albarracin CA, et al. Chromium picolinate and biotin combination improves glucose metabolism in treated, uncontrolled overweight to obese patients with type 2 diabetes. *Diabetes/Metabolism Research & Reviews.* 24(1):41-51, 2008.

Alschuler, Lise and Karolyn A. Gazella. *Definitive Guide to Cancer.* Berkeley, CA: Celestial Arts, 2007.

Anukam KC, et al. Clinical study comparing probiotic Lactobacillus GR-1 and RC-14 with metronidazole vaginal gel to treat symptomatic bacterial vaginosis. *Microbes and Infection.* 8(12-13):2772-6, 2006.

Brown AD, et al. Effects of cardiovascular fitness and cerebral blood flow on cognitive outcomes in older women. *Neurobiology of Aging.* 2008.

Cao H, et al. Cinnamon extract and polyphenols affect the expression of tristetraprolin, insulin receptor, and glucose transporter 4 in moust 3T3-L1 adipocytes. *Archives of Biochemistry and Biophysics.* 459:214-222, published online Jan 2007.

Du X, et al. Oral benfotiamine plus alpha-lipoic acid normalizes complication-causing pathways in type 1 diabetes. *Diabetologia.* Jul 29, 2008.

Eby, Myra Michelle, and Karolyn A. Gazella. *Return To Beautiful Skin,* Laguna Beach, CA: Basic Health Publications, 2008.

Fuchs, Nan Kathyrn. The New Way to Stop Gums from Bleeding and Save Your Teeth. *Women's Health Letter,* September 2007.

Geier MS, et al. Inflammatory bowel disease: Current insights into pathogenesis and new therapeutic options; probiotics, prebiotics, and synbiotics. *International Journal of Food Microbiology.* 115(1):1-11, 2007.

Geier MS, et al. Probiotics, prebiotics and synbiotics: A role in chemoprevention for colorectal cancer? *Cancer Biology & Therapy.* 5(10):1265-9, 2006.

Head KA, Jurenka JS. Crohn's disease—pathophysiology and conventional and alternative treatment options. *Alternative Medicine Review.* 9(4), 2004.

Hughes VL, Hillier SL. Microbiologic characteristics of lactobacillus products used for colonization of the vagina. *Obstetrics and Gynecology.* 75(2):244-8, 1990.

Jones J. What is the role of bacteria in cancer carcinogenesis? *Journal of the National Cancer Institute.* 92(21):1713, 2000.

Margolis DJ, et al. Effects of antibiotics on the oropharyngeal flora in patients with acne. *Archives of Dermatology.* 139(4):467-471, 2003.

McFarland LV. Meta-analysis of probiotics for the prevention of traveler's diarrhea. *Travel Medicine and Infectious Disease.* 5(2):97-105, 2007.

Najm WI, et al. S-adenosyl methionine (SAMe) versus celecoxib for the treatment of osteoarthritis symptoms: A double-blind cross-over trial. *BMC Musculoskeletal Disorders.* 5:6, 2004.

Onderdonk AB. Probiotics for women's health. *Journal of Clinical Gastroenterology.* 40(3):256-9, 2006.

Pescatore, Fred. *The Allergy & Asthma Cure.* Somerset, NJ: Wiley & Sons, 2003.

Quigley EM. Probiotics in irritable bowel syndrome: An immunomodulatory strategy? *Journal of the American College of Nutrition.* 26(6):684S-90S, 2007.

Rafter, J, et al. Dietary synbiotics reduce cancer risk factors in polypectomized and colon cancer patients. *American Journal of Clinical Nutrition*. 85(2):488-96, 2007.

Reid G, et al. Probiotic Lactobacillus dose required to restore and maintain a normal vaginal flora. *FEMS Immunology and Medical Microbiology*. 32(1):37-41, 2001.

Sanders ME. Consideration for use of probiotic bacteria to modulate human health. *Journal of Nutrition*. 130(2S Suppl):384S-390S, 2000.

Singer GM, Geohas J. The effect of chromium picolinate and biotin supplementation on glycemic control in poorly controlled patients with Type 2 diabetes mellitus: A placebo-controlled, double-blinded, randomized trial. *Diabetes Technology & Therapeutics*. 8(6), 2006.

Spiller P. Review article: Probiotics and prebiotics in irritable bowel syndrome (IBS). *Alimentary Pharmacology & Therapeutics*. 28(4):385-96, 2008.

Teughels W, et al. Guiding periodontal pocket recolonization: a proof of concept. *Journal of Dental Research*. 86(11):1078-1082, 2007.

Valdoria HT. The effect of probiotics in the treatment of acute non-bloody diarrhea in infants aged 3 to 24 Months. Research findings presented by Hazel T Valdoria, MD, at the First Congress of Asian Society for Pediatric Research, Nov 2005.

Wilhelm SM, et al. Effectiveness of probiotics in the treatment of irritable bowel syndrome. *Pharmacotherapy*. 28(4):496-505, 2008.

Chapter 11

http://www.nlm.nih.gov/medlineplus/healthtopics_a.html

Alschuler, Lise and Karolyn A. Gazella. *Definitive Guide to Cancer*. Berkeley, CA: Celestial Arts, 2007.

Barnett KJ. The effects of a poor night sleep on mood, cognitive, autonomic and electrophysiological measure. *Journal of Integrative Neuroscience*. 7(3):405-20, 2008.

Diop L, et al. Probiotic food supplement reduces stress-induced gastrointestinal symptoms in volunteers: A double-blind, placebo-controlled, randomized trial. *Nutrition Research*. 28(1):1-5, 2008.

Gittleman, Ann Louise. *The Gut Flush Plan*, New York:Avery Publishing, 2008.

Kleiner SM. Water: An essential but overlooked nutrient. *Journal of The American Dietetic Association*. 99(2):200-206, 1999.

Patel SR, et al. The association between sleep duration and obesity in older adults. *International Journal of Obesity*. 32(12):1825-34, 2008.

Pescatore, Fred. *The Allergy & Asthma Cure*. Somerset, NJ: Wiley & Sons, 2003.

Pescatore, Fred. *The Hamptons Diet*. Somerset, NJ: Wiley & Sons, 2004.

Roth, T. Prevalence, associated risks, and treatment patterns of insomnia. *Journal of Clinical Psychiatry*. 66(suppl 9):10-13, 2005.

Sadeghniiat-Haghighi K, et al. Efficacy and hypnotic effects of melatonin in shift-work nurses: Double-blind, placebo-controlled crossover trial. *Journal of Circadian Rhythms*. 6:10, 2008.

Vgontzas AN, et al. Chronic insomnia is associated with nyctohemeral activation of the hypothalamic-pituitary-adrenal axis: Clinical implications. *Journal of Clinical Endocrinology and Metabolism*. 86(8):3787-3794, 2001.

Wade A, Downie S. Prolonged-release melatonin for the treatment of insomnia in patients over 55 years. *Expert Opinion on Investigational Drugs*. 17(10):1567-72, 2008.

Walker MP. Sleep-dependent memory processing. *Harvard Review of Psychiatry*. 16(5):287-98, 2008.

Winkelman JW, et al. Reduced brain GABA in primary insomnia: preliminary data from 4T proton magnetic resonance spectroscopy (1H-MRS). *Sleep*. 31(11):1499-506, 2008.

Xie Q, et al. Inhibition of acrylamide toxicity in mice by three dietary constituents. *Journal of Agricultural and Food Chemistry*. 56(15):6054-60, 2008.

INDEX

Acid indigestion, 169
Acne, 17, 144–45
Aging
  bacterial imbalance and, 122
  dementia and, 157
  sleep deprivation and, 204
Allergies
  to antibiotics, 13
  causes of, 146
  description of, 146
  GMOs and, 108, 109
  treatment of, 146–47
All-nighters, 205
Alzheimer's disease, 130, 132, 157
Amino acids, 86
Amoxicillin, 13
Anthrax, 20, 83
Antibiotics
  allergies to, 13
  broad-spectrum, 14–15
  development of new, 13
  discovery of, 12–13
  in food and water supply, 15
  livestock industry's use of, 15–16,
    41, 54–55
  natural alternatives to, 23
  overuse of, 14–15, 21–22

  prevalence of, 13
  probiotics after use of, 77
  resistance to, 13–14, 16–17, 19,
    54–55
  side effects of, 14–15
  soil-based organisms and, 83
Antimicrobial products, 22, 24, 52
Antioxidants, 136, 138, 140
Arginine, 86
Arthritis, 148–49
Aspartame, 84
Autism, 91, 122
Autoimmune conditions, 138

Bacillus, 83
Bacillus anthracis, 20
Bacillus licheniformis, 83
Bacteria. See also Bacterial imbalance;
  Beneficial bacteria; Probiotics
  antibiotic resistance in, 13–14,
    16–17, 19, 54–55
  characteristics of, 28
  communication by, 32–34, 40–41
  communities of, 29
  definition of, 17
  discovery of, 8–9
  fear of, 74, 97

first, 8
harmful, 10–11, 20, 38, 39, 45–46,
     48–51
initial exposure to, at birth, 36
origin of the word, 9
prevalence of, in the human body, 1,
     8, 27–28, 29
reducing exposure to, 48–51
shapes of, 27
size of, 28
species and strains of, 28–29
viruses vs., 17, 19, 21
Bacterial imbalance (dysbiosis)
antibiotic use and, 14–15
causes of, 39
correcting, 189
diagnosis of, 40
disease and, 193–94, 210
effects of, 3, 35–36, 38, 40, 122,
     193–94
leaky gut syndrome and, 120
mental health and, 137
quiz on, 37
symptoms of, 48
Bacterioides theta, 85
Beneficial bacteria. See also Probiotics
competitive exclusion and, 34, 120
importance of, 2, 8, 35
supporting, 67–69
tasks performed by, 34–35, 36–37,
     61–64
Benign prostatic hyperplasia (BPH), 181
Berberine, 23
Bifidobacterium, 79, 80, 84, 85
Biotin, 64
Bipolar disorder, 137
Body mass index (BMI), 130, 131
Bone mineral density (BMD) test, 179
Botulism, 10, 20
Bowel movements, 122
Breast cancer, 19
Breathing exercises, 200–201
Brucella abortus, 20
Bubonic plague, 10

Canadine, 23
Cancer. See also individual cancers
causes of, 150
description of, 150
obesity and, 130
prevalence of, 132
treatment of, 150–51
Candida albicans, 23
Cardiovascular disease. See Heart
     disease
Celiac disease, 152–53
Centrifugation, 94–95
CFUs (colony forming units), 77–80
Chemical exposure, 124
Children
autism in, 91
diabetes in, 159
hygiene and, 18, 50
probiotics for, 76, 135
Chlamydia, 23
Chloramphenicol, 13
Cholera, 10, 20
Chronic fatigue syndrome, 137
Clindamycin, 17
Clostridium botulinum, 10, 20
Clostridium difficile (C. diff), 17
Cold, common, 14, 21
Colitis, 154
Colon
bacteria in, 116, 118
cancer, 47, 151
importance of, 115
pH of, 82
Colonoscopy, 47
Competitive exclusion, 34, 120
Constipation, 122
Corynebacterium diphtheria, 23
Crohn's disease, 155–56

Dairy-based probiotics, 91
Death, leading causes of, 132
Dehydration, 198–99
Deinococcus radiodurans, 123
Dementia, 130, 157–58

Dermatitis, 166
Detoxification, 122, 124, 126
Diabetes, 130, 132–36, 159–61
Diagnostic tests, 46–47
Diarrhea, 162–63. *See also* Traveler's
  diarrhea
Diet
  fats in, 65–67
  fiber in, 63
  importance of, 194–98
  rotating, with seasons, 68
  standard American, 65, 159
  sugar in, 65, 129, 134, 138
Dietary supplements. *See* Supplements
Digestion
bacteria and, 62–64
elimination and detoxification, 122,
  124, 126
importance of, 126–27
leaky gut syndrome, 118–22
process of, 116, 117
Diplococcus pneumonia, 23
Disease prevention
  bacterial balance and, 193–94, 210–11
  diet and, 194–98
  exercise and, 202–3
  hydration and, 198–99
  immune system and, 136, 138–40
  inflammation control and, 140–41
  insulin resistance control and, 134–36
  lifestyle factors and, 129
  obesity reduction and, 130–34
  sleep and, 204–8
  supplements and, 208–10
Diverticulitis, 164
Dr. Ohhira's Essential Living Oils, 67
Dr. Ohhira's Probiotics 12 PLUS, 60, 84,
  170, 171, 189
Dysbiosis, 40, 118. *See also* Bacterial
  imbalance

E. coli, 10, 16, 20, 39, 49, 51, 165
Eczema, 166
Elimination, 122, 124, 126

Endoscopy, 47
Enterococcus faecalis TH10, 93, 99, 105
Enzymes, 85–86
ERCP (endoscopic retrograde
  cholangiopancreatography), 47
Escherichia coli. See E. coli
Essential fatty acids (EFAs), 65–67, 209
Eubiosis, 118
Exercise, 68, 125, 200, 202–3

Fats, 65–67
Fermentation, 11–12, 58, 82, 84, 93, 95,
  100–101
Fiber, 63
Flax, 61, 67
Fleming, Sir Alexander, 12–13
Flu, 18, 19, 21, 132, 167–68
Food. *See also* Diet
  choosing, 194–98
  fiber in, 63
  genetically modified, 107–10
  organic, 41, 55
  poisoning, 10, 20, 49
Free radicals, 136, 140
Freeze-drying, 94
French fries, 195
Fructooligosaccharides (FOS), 84–85

GABA (gamma-aminobutyric acid), 206
GALT (gut-association lymphoid tissue),
  133, 139
Garlic, 23
Gastroenteritis, 167–68
Gastroenterology, 101–2, 104
Gastroesophageal reflux disease
  (GERD), 169–70
Germ theory, 11–12
Giardiasis, 51
Gingivitis, 171–72
Gittleman, Ann Louise, 105
Glucose, 134
Gluten, 152–53
GMOs (genetically modified
  organisms), 107–11

Golden Rice, 110
Goldenseal, 23
Gottfried Ehrenberg, Christian, 9
Greens, 196
Gum disease. *See* Gingivitis

Hand-washing tips, 50
Healthcare, future of, 211
Heartburn, 169
Heart disease, 130, 132, 173–74
Helicobacter pylori, 38, 49, 123, 151, 186, 196–97
Histidine, 86
Human Microbiome Project, 30–32, 42–43, 89, 90, 102, 105–7
Huntington's disease, 157
Hydrastine, 23
Hydration, 198–99
Hygiene, 18, 49–51

Immune system
    digestive tract and, 62, 133, 139
    free radicals and, 136
    function of, 62, 136
    inflammation and, 140–41
    probiotics and, 133, 139
    stimulating, 138–39
Inflammation, 140–41
Inflammatory bowel disease. *See* Colitis; Crohn's disease
Influenza. *See* Flu
Insomnia, 69, 204–8
Insulin resistance, 134–36
Irritable bowel syndrome (IBS), 175–76
Isoleucine, 86

Kidney disease, 132
Krensky, Alan M., 31, 42–43, 105–7

Lactobacillus acidophilus, 79, 81
Lactobacillus brevis, 79
Lactobacillus bulgaricus, 79
Lactobacillus casei, 79
Lactobacillus fermentum, 139

Lactobacillus rhamnosus, 80, 90
Lactose intolerance, 91
Leaky gut syndrome, 118–22
Legionella pneumophila, 10, 20, 39
Legionnaire's disease, 10, 20, 39
Leprosy, 10
Leucine, 86
Listeria monocytogenes, 10
Liver
    disease, 126, 177–78
    function of, 122, 124
Lung cancer, 150
Lysine, 86

Macadamia nut oil, 66
Massage, 200
McNeil Consumer Healthcare, 52
Meat
    antibiotics in, 15–16, 41, 54–55
    organic, 41, 55
Meditation, 200
Melatonin, 206
Mental health, 137
Metchnikoff, Elie, 12, 27
Methicillin, 22
Methionine, 86
Methylcobalamin, 207
Microbiome, definition of, 30
Microflora, definition of, 28
Milk, mother's, 81
Miso, 58
Monounsaturated fats, 66
MRSA (methicillin-resistant *Staphylococcus aureus*), 11, 19, 22, 39
Muscle relaxation, progressive, 200
Mycobacterium leprae, 10
Mycobacterium tuberculosis, 20
Mycobacterium vaccae, 137

National Center for Complementary and Alternative Medicine (NCCAM), 60
National Institutes of Health (NIH), 30–32, 42, 89, 105–7

Obesity, 59, 130–34
Obsessive-compulsive disorder, 137
Occult blood analysis, 47
Ohhira, Iichiroh, 58, 60, 78, 81, 82, 86, 92–93, 95, 97–101, 165, 180, 183, 185, 189
Oils, 66–67
Oligosaccharides, 81, 84
Olive oil, 66–67
Organic meat and poultry, 41, 55
Osteoarthritis, 148–49
Osteoporosis, 179–80

Pandemics, 10
Parkinson's disease, 157
Pasteur, Louis Jean, 11–12, 94
Pelton, Ross, 104–5
Penicillin, 12–13, 17
Peptic ulcers. *See* Ulcers
Phagocytosis, 12
Phenylananine, 86
Physical activity, 68, 125, 200, 202–3
Pneumonia, 20, 132
Polyunsaturated fats, 66
Positive attitude, 201
Poultry
    antibiotics in, 15–16, 41, 54–55
    organic, 41, 55
Prebiotics, 59, 82, 84–85, 194–95
Probiotics. *See also* Beneficial bacteria
    as alternative to antibiotics, 23
    bacterial strains in, 79, 80–81
    bacterial viability of, 78–81, 89
    benefits of, 60–61, 189
    CFUs and, 77–80
    for children, 76, 135
    choosing, 89
    constipation and, 122
    dairy-based, 91
    definition of, 27, 58
    in food, 88, 197
    future of, 97–107, 111–12
    genetically modified, 110–11
    high potency, 78–79

immune system and, 133, 139
individuals needing, 74–77
leaky gut syndrome and, 120
mental health and, 137
misconceptions about, 103
popularity of, 60, 87–88
prebiotics and, 82, 84–85, 194–95
production of, 93–95, 99–101
quality of, 89, 102–3, 104, 105
quiz on, 75
safety of, 80
scientific research on, 89–90, 92
in skin and dental products, 197
soil-based organisms as, 83
weight loss and, 59, 133
Prostate disorders, 181
Psoriasis, 182–83
Purell hand sanitizer, 52

Quigley, Eamonn, 30, 59, 101–4, 111, 176
Quorum sensing, 33

Reid, Gregor, 58, 64, 104, 188
Relaxation techniques, 200–201
Respiratory diseases, 130, 132
Rheumatoid arthritis, 148–49

SAD (standard American diet), 65, 159
Salmonella, 10, 20, 49
Salmonella typhi, 20, 23
Sanitizers, 22, 24, 52
Saturated fats, 65
Schizophrenia, 137
Septicemia, 132
Sigmoidoscopy, 47
Silymarin, 126
Skin cancer, 150
Sleep, 69, 204–8
Small intestine
    bacteria in, 116, 118
    function of, 118
Soil-based organisms (SBOs), 83
Spontaneous generation, 11

Staph infection, 10, 11, 19, 22
Staphylococcus aureus, 10, 20. *See also*
   MRSA
Stomach
   acid in, 123
   bacteria in, 123
   cancer, 151
   flu, 167–68
   ulcers, 123, 186–87
Stool analysis, 47
Strep throat, 10, 19, 20, 21
Streptococcus pneumoniae, 20
Streptococcus pyogenes, 10
Streptomycin, 13
Stress
   insomnia and, 205
   reduction, 68, 200–201
Stroke, 130, 132, 157
Sugar, 65, 129, 134, 138
Sulfonamides, 13
Superbugs
   antibiotic overuse and, 15–16
   definition of, 15
Supplements. *See also* Probiotics
   buying, 209
   disease prevention and, 208–10
   sleep and, 206–7
   stress and, 201
Sweeteners, artificial, 84
Swine flu, 18
Synbiotics, 86
Systemic illnesses, 45–46

Tempeh, 58
Tetracycline, 13
Theanine, 206–7
Threonin, 86
Tomatoes, 109–10
Trans fats, 66
Traveler's diarrhea, 184–85
Treponema pallidum, 137
Tryptophan, 86, 206
Tuberculosis, 20
Typhoid fever, 20

Ulcers, 123, 186–87
Ultrafiltration, 95

Vaginitis, 188–89
Valine, 86
Van Leeuwenhoek, Antony, 8–9
Vibrio cholerae, 20, 23
Vibrio vulnificus, 10
Viruses
   antibiotics and, 21
   bacteria vs., 17, 19, 21
   definition of, 17
   preventing spread of, 18
Visualization, 200
Vitamins
   A, 124, 138
   B12, 116, 207
   C, 124, 138, 163
   D, 138
   E, 66, 138
   K, 64

Waist circumference, 130, 132–33
Water
   antibiotics in, 15, 51
   bacteria in, 51
   bottled, 51
   importance of, 198–99
   toxins in, 51, 199
Weight loss, 32, 59, 133

Yersinia pestis, 10
Yogurt, 80

ABOUT THE AUTHORS

Fred Pescatore, MD, is one of the key spokespersons for healthy living. His latest New York Times best-selling book, *The Hampton's Diet*, and *The Hampton's Diet Cookbook*, combines the Mediterranean lifestyle with the palates of Americans emphasizing a whole foods approach to health and weight management. He lectures around the world and has been seen on such televisions shows as, Today, The View, AM Canada, and many others. He is a correspondent for *Women's World*, *First for Women*, *In Touch*, *US Weekly* and *Life & Style* magazines. Dr. Pescatore is the co-host of New Vitality Live, a nationally syndicated weekly radio show. He is also a member of the American College for the Advancement of Medicine, the President of the International and American Association of Clinical Nutritionists and the National Association of Medical Broadcasters. Dr. Pescatore has also authored *Feed Your Kids Well*, *Thin for Good*, and *The Allergy and Asthma Cure*. Please visit him at www.hamptonsdiet.com or www.drpescatore.com for more information.

Karolyn A. Gazella is a veteran health writer and the co-author of the *Definitive Guide to Cancer* and *Return to Beautiful Skin*. She is also the publisher and editor of an online journal and content website for healthcare professionals, www.naturalmedicinejournal.com. She is the managing editor of the *Healthy Living Guide Series*, an educational booklet program available through *Better Nutrition* magazine. She has written hundreds of articles on the topic of natural health for a variety of magazines. For more information, visit www.karolyngazella.com.